T1 INCREDIBLE POWER OF INSPIRATION

Creating the Life You Yearn for

Jenifer Zetlan

For permission requests, please contact the publisher at:

Mango Publishing Group
2850 Douglas Road, 3rd Floor
Coral Gables, FL 33134 USA
info@mango.bz

For special orders, quantity sales, course adoptions and corporate sales,
please email the publisher at sales@mango.bz. For trade and wholesale
sales, please contact Ingram Publisher Services at customer.service@
ingramcontent.com or +1.800.509.4887.

The Incredible Power of Inspiration: Creating the Life You Yearn For

Library of Congress Cataloging
ISBN: (print) 978-1-63353-627-2, (ebook) 978-1-63353-628-9
Library of Congress Control Number: 2017955627
BISAC category code: OCC010000, BODY, MIND & SPIRIT / Mindfulness &
Meditation

Printed in the United States of America

to

the memory of Ruth, the mother of my inspiration

and

Michael, the greatest seedling of all

TABLE OF CONTENTS

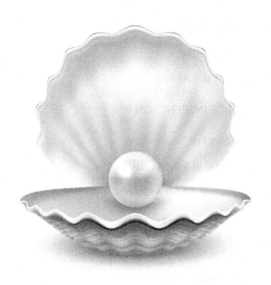

INTRODUCTION

"And now here is my secret, a very simple secret: It is only with the heart that one can see rightly; what is essential is invisible to the eye."

–Antoine de Saint-Exupéry, The Little Prince

∿

"Don't be pushed around by the fears in your mind. Be led by the dreams in your heart."

–Roy T. Bennett, The Light in the Heart

Inspiration is a powerful thing. It drives us towards new ideas and new goals, and it helps us solve life's mysteries. Many of us love a great mystery, one that begins with an inexplicable event that none of the characters can quite grasp – but the Big Event leaves in its wake an equally "Big Question." The question draws us forward in search of clues, and along that path we make discoveries large and small. Sometimes resolution resounds with a bang (for better or worse!), sometimes it's a sleeper, and sometimes the resolution offers us a startling surprise that leads to a crescendo and a victorious end. You just never know, but the ride is fantastic!

When I was a young child, my father died inexplicably at the age of thirty-seven, leaving behind at least two Big Questions for me and my family. For my mother, her big question was: "How do I raise two young children by myself?" For my brother, it was: "Will I also die young?" For me, at the age of three, the Big Question was: "What happened to Daddy?"

Like all good mysteries, I couldn't understand why mortal illness struck my father down at such a young age. I began to follow the clues about wellness and about what may have happened to him. I employed my father's premature death and my mother's pure grief and grit to propel me towards living a long, healthy, and vibrant life. I sought out heart-healthy distance running and the study of psychology – I wanted to know why people are the way that they are, and how people may best reach their potentials. The study of psychology morphed into science, then into philosophy, and finally ripened into spirituality. Throughout my life, solving this mystery has been a propelling inspiration.

After four decades of study in psychology, philosophy, comparative religion, and health and wellness, I was inspired to deepen my knowledge and decided to study yoga. My yoga practice opened up many new mysteries that inspired me to seek further. Through my inquires into deepening yoga practice, I began to experience the linkages between diverse areas of our lives. I began to research Hindu texts from 1500 BC, Talmudic mystical teachings from the oral tradition from the early Common Era, and contemporary-inspired writings of Christianity. I studied physics and anatomy; I tasted biology and neuroscience – I kept exploring different disciplines, finding strikingly similar patterns of questions, quests, and queries. A discovery in one field inspired more learning about ourselves and our world.

The authors I read continued to inspire me – I saw them as life's adventurers, forging new ground as they sought answers to their own Big Questions. They embarked upon quests and followed clues; they queried, then queried some more. Their lives were intensely infused with passion and curiosity. They often took the apparently mundane, taken-for-granted parts of their lives and turned them into something much bigger, more important – one might even say more sacred – phenomena. Mozart liked a good tune, Plato loved a good question, and modern day astrophysicist Neil deGrasse Tyson loves to stargaze.

Looking through the rear-view mirror of inquiry over my lifetime (so far), I have come to believe that in the mysteries of our lives, there are two key elements which guide you: inspiration and wellness. Each discipline I studied, in whatever technical language that it was presented, delivered that message consistently: "All of life is an evolving grand mystery, so do what inspires you and be fit, or well enough, to do it."

The Starting Point: Life is a Mystery. I am constantly humbled by the mystery that lies at the cutting edge of all things, the Big Questions that rest on their horizon, and the "enfold-ment" of what might emerge next. Early in my youth, people were the greatest mystery to me. We "were all people," yet so different from one another. Why? What are feelings? Where do they come from? Why are weird people weird? Why are healthy people healthy? Then there was music. Where does music come from? How does someone hear music in their head and then compose a piece of music? In the world of work, how do companies work with so many ("unique") people involved? In aerospace, how are ideas for spacecraft conceived? How do people manage their relationships to bring a design to life? How does a single inspiration alter the course of history?

We, the conceivers of our own reality, have always been, and will always be, the Greatest Mystery of all – to me.

We each have our own "Great Mysteries." Those things we yearn to know about and that we would love to dedicate much of our time to in exploration. What tickles your imagination? What calls you to action, to explore and expand?

The Constant: Do what inspires you. We are all aware of people who were inspired and changed the world. Einstein was inspired to explore the universe through "thought experiments." Patanjali, a Hindu scholar circa 1500 BC, was inspired to explore the transience of objects like a clay pot – or our own bodies. He urged us to conquer the mysteries of our mental flotsam in the depths of our own consciousness. Plato egged us on to "look from within" and set the model for the modern philosopher. Neil deGrasse Tyson was inspired to explore the mysteries of the universe and engages millions of people across the globe to do the same.

The message? Inspiration is for us all. When you uncover your mysteries, face them with compassion and curiosity, and ask your Big Questions. You will gain the freedom to explore, to engage your imagination – to dance to the beat of your own drum, to laugh, and to grow as if no one is watching...and to always love. Do what inspires you; do what floats your boat; do it with abandon.

The Requirement: Wellness. There is only one requirement to delving into your greatest mystery and living an inspired life, and that is Wellness. We all yearn to live vibrant and meaningful lives, to embrace our own mysteries, but without wellness it is difficult, if not nearly impossible. When you are ensnared in the treacherous undertow of illness, or of grief, or of entrenched emotional habits, these become the focus of your life. Pain, struggle, and illness are the "vacuous siphons" of vitality. They drain our mental, emotional, and physical health, and direct our energy in negative directions into deeper downward spirals.

Wellness is a choice; we choose wellness every moment of every day. We choose healthy diet and exercise, or not. We choose to have healthy relationships, or choose to remain in poor ones. We choose to honor our feelings for the information they contain, or we suppress them and allow them to gain momentum under the skin. We choose ethical thinking, or live out of delusion. We acknowledge the mystery of spirit, or cap it off with cynicism or boredom.

However you may conceive your life to be right now – today – please understand that you are in the driver's seat. You have created the life that you are living today, and you will create the life that you will live tomorrow, and the day after. Whether or not you embrace your greatest mysteries, whether you ignite your inspiration and choose wellness or instead hole up and constrict the human experience that is you, know that you are the chooser.

There is much to learn about being _you_. Discover and embrace your own Great Mysteries: ask the Big Questions, truly grasp what it is that you yearn for, and graciously allow the Way of your inspiration to propel you forward. All questions will be answered simply because they have been asked; relentlessly live into your inspiration. Wellness, you will find, is the byproduct of living an inspired life.

I am writing this book for all of us. I want to document what I have come to believe helps us to understand the Grand Mystery of being human, to embody the essence of the inspired life that I yearn for (and am always creating), and to share my experience with my son and granddaughter.

I am also writing this book for you, the reader. I want to share how to create the life that you yearn for, to jump into the mystery that is you and live into your inspiration with bold anticipation and joy. I call this experience your "Frontier Adventure," allowing your inspiration to pierce through the edges of your everyday life and forge new pathways that are uniquely yours. I deeply hope that you will share what you learn with others and leave new footholds for those behind you.

In gratitude of the Great Mysteries that bring forth our inspiration,

– J. K. S. Zetlan
2017

NOTE TO THE READER

This is a book of spiritual adventure towards living a more inspired life. It is written to provide new and modern insights along a path that has been traveled for centuries by spiritual masters, philosophers, physicists, psychologists, doctors, and ordinary people like us.

The amount of research and discourse about our spirituality fills racks of library shelves, material that is often too dense to absorb. In this book, I have taken the reader on a spiritual "hike" through a forest of information in a manner intended to inform our everyday experience in an easily relatable manner. The story is both a spiritual tale and a guide for what we experience as we grow into older, wiser, and more playful adults. It is a whimsical tale that delves into intimate and deeply personal experiences we have all had, or will have.

The book is divided into three parts:

Part I addresses our mind–body experience in a day-to-day environment. It addresses the concept of everyone's core beliefs and develops a better understanding of what well-being entails. It explores how we make choices that propel us forward toward living an inspired life. Tools are provided to help the reader understand emotions and behavior so we can journey well beyond the emotional baggage we have all collected throughout our lives, from childhood until now.

Part II explores the bottlenecks and debris that get in the way of inspired thinking. The reader learns specific strategies to break through deeply ingrained habits that hold back inspired thought and how to let go of outdated life stories. This Part provides the tools to release the grip of the deepest fears that prevent us from moving forward beyond what might be possible, challenging thoughts about limitations.

Part III shifts gears and takes a sharp right turn to enable the reader to navigate the mental and spiritual corridors of our lives. While Parts I and II focused primarily on releasing ourselves from habitual and self-limiting lives, Part III takes us on a journey of inspiration and deeper meaning. While Parts I and II are a guide to becoming an expert "human being," Part III enables the reader to realize the power of inspiration through self-reflection and spiritual mastery.

We all travel a path on life's journey. Some of us travel further, and some of us get stuck on the "path of our own doing." It is this author's intention to enable the reader to clear some of the debris and to provide access to the power of inspiration.

Happy Trails!

— Jenifer Zetlan

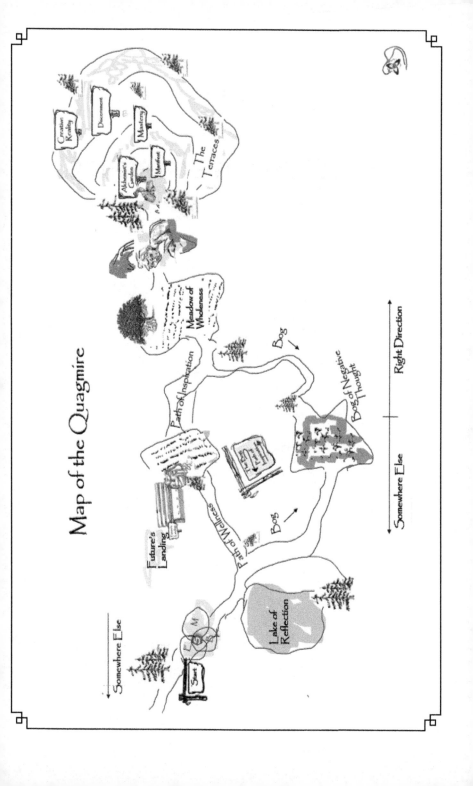

PART I

THE ALCHEMY OF EXPERIENCE

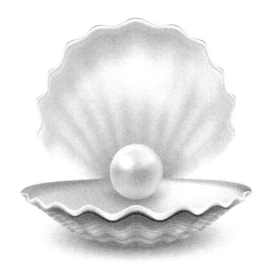

∞

Chapter 1

~

Living into Our Beliefs

Stop...Look...And listen!

—Mrs. Fisher,
Kindergarten Teacher, Aurora, CO, 1956

"Remember that wherever your heart is, there
you will find your treasure."

—Paulo Coelho, The Alchemist

Imagine that your own *Book of Life Past* lay before you, inexplicably appearing in carefully fashioned leather binding, your name painstakingly engraved in gold-leaf letters on its rubbed brown leather cover, a sweet image of a dancer delicately embossed beneath your name. Inscribed on each worn parchment page is a tender accounting of your years gone by. It may look like a sacred text, tantalizing to the touch and filled with carefully selected moments lifted from the many years of your life. Within the chronicled pages are your own cherished moments, whether they detail a secret recounting of your joys, your deepest wishes, or your most troubled times. All those precious "Notes to Self," each one carefully selected to remind you of the ups and downs of your life, your hard-earned lessons, your personally crafted life's philosophy, and perhaps even some suggestions for your future self.

Imagine that you randomly open to any page in your *Book of Life Past*. Even if a bit of trepidation or hesitation may cause you pause, you open the book with compassion, knowing your journey has been sometimes sweet or arduous at times, perhaps with periods of relative calm as your spirit drew respite from life's currents. As you breathe these moments that are uniquely yours into your heart, you can see they contain your life's Greatest Mysteries. On some pages they were recorded outright, and on others weighty messages lay hidden between the lines. Perhaps you chance upon a life-changing event, or a fresh and exhilarating experience. Maybe a heart-breaking drama is unfolding, or perhaps a question remains unresolved. This collection of experience is you.

Written within your mysterious chronicles are the moments that brought you forward into your life as it is today. Born of your life's exploration and gradual expansion, you can see your own Great Mysteries through the perspective of time. Breathe deeply: you have arrived at the very center of you; the Knower, the Wise Soul, the observer and source of your own yearning and inspiration that carries with it the power to create worlds. Life is the Grandest Mystery of all, and it begs us to wrestle with the Big Questions.

In this book, you will learn how to adventure into your own Great Mysteries, embrace the Big Questions that contain the sweet nectar of yearning, and master the Process of Inspiration. You will learn how to consciously access your native inspiration and free yourself to imagine into being the life that you yearn for. You will find ways to become more grounded that will help strengthen your esteem and resilience as you learn to hold the course and follow your dreams. It is my hope that this book will compel you to explore the Great Mysteries of your life, devour their intrigue, and chart your path forward through practical application. Jump into your own Mysteries with abandon, simmer with the Big Questions, and use the simple tools and exercises in this book as your guide.

Reverie Interrupted

Phone rings. Texts arrive, heralding the appointment you are already late for. Your reverie in the *Book of Life Past* is so easily interrupted. At the very moment you can almost touch the horizon of your inspired self, the buzz of your phone startles you out of your dream. With anxiety and a quick shot of adrenaline, your "hurry up" crawls across your skin as you jump into action. You are angry at yourself for your moment of self-absorption, because "real life" calls. You pause to take one last glimpse at your *Book of Life Past*, only to find that it has vanished as inexplicably as it materialized.

Perhaps you wonder, "What just happened?" It felt real at the moment, but in the flash of an interruption, the experience dissolved like a dream upon waking. And like a dream, the experience is difficult to recapture, as if it never happened. This experience leads to a Big Question: "How will I ever recover that sense of awareness and awe, of meaning, of deep yearning and electrified inspiration?"

You must become an "Alchemist" of your own experience – working to master the powerful currents alive within you. Alchemy, from medieval times, is described as a transformation of base metals into gold. It was considered an elemental practice and was believed to extend one's longevity. In this book we will revere Alchemy through a more philosophical lens as we consider it in the framework of being a deeply human process – one of self exploration, discovery, imagination, and mastery, with the conscious intention of transforming our hectic lives into golden quests. I believe that understanding the Alchemy of our own experience will extend one's well-being and longevity.

Authentic inspiration resides at our very core and is an unwilling participant in turbulent, restrictive, or oppressive environments – internal or external. Natural inspiration, especially in its early stages, feels fragile to the novice Alchemist. It needs supportive space within your own heart and mind, allowing it to flow forth safely. Drama is a deal breaker, at least temporarily, as torrential currents crash against sensitive desire. But if we learn how to navigate our inner lives, we can harness the power of inspiration and live into our dreams. This is the Alchemy of Inspiration!

The Alchemy of Inspiration

At a very general level we are all aware that we have some type of internal chemistry; we experience a variety of feelings, thoughts, and moods that are apt to change minute by minute or day to day. The flow of our lives is similar to the movement of the ocean, with currents, undertows, transient flotsam, waves that tickle the shore and play, and waves with deep undertows. The currents have unpredictable vortexes that swirl in ways that are mysterious to the casual observer, but are understood and predictable to seasoned oceanographers who are studied in the ways of the sea.

So, too, we are bristling oceans of physical and non-physical matter. Like the ocean, we have intellectual currents, emotional undertows, moods that tickle and invite us into play, and a deep potential for ruthless joy and inspiration.

Through becoming adept with the Alchemy of experience, we can tap into and harness our own experiences to better navigate our internal oceans – our internal dynamics and unique chemistry. Once trained, we can better understand our feelings, create moods, harness our intellect, and reach the pinnacle of inspiration – that place in all of us where we feel fully alive, where we ingest the world with ravenous curiosity and unapologetically imagine our dreams into being. Living into Inspiration is our journey!

We all have the ability to become masterful alchemists who are studied in the ways of our own internal chemistry. A novice oceanographer sees only a sea with powerful waves and cyclic ebb and flow of the tides; he or she knows of potential peril or pleasure only from reading nearby signposts. However, once studied, the oceanographer gains an intuitive mastery over the knowledge of the seas, above and below the surface, and can recognize minute changes in pressure, currents, topography, and temperature. Skilled sailors use the knowledge of the oceanographer to become artists at altering their course in the face of peril or quickly changing direction to explore new territory. They are alchemists of the seas, engaging experience, science, intuition, and knowledge to best steer their course.

As novice alchemists of experience, we know a little bit about our physical form and movement and are aware that there is an endless streaming cacophony of thoughts and feelings racing about in our minds. However, once we become studied in the currents of our experience and how our energies ebb and flow, we will understand much more about our physical, emotional, and intellectual makeup and become more attuned to small changes in our internal and external environments. As we become more knowledgeable about our own unique mechanics, we will be able to masterfully innovate and create both our experience and the lives that we deeply yearn for. We will be able to adventure into our Grand Mysteries with confidence and engage science, intuition, and knowledge to access our deepest inspiration. We will watch as the awesome power of inspiration flows forth – if, that is, we can find enough moments in the day to exit the frenetically paced quagmire of our daily lives to transform our reveries into realities.

Life in the Quagmire

We live in the twenty-first century...life in the fast lane...we have careers to build, relationships to maintain, we have rent to pay, food to prepare, places to be, and worries about how to get there. Many of us have kids to raise, parents to support, and seemingly never enough sleep. We have an overload of data and good advice we can access, but it takes so much effort to sort through and manage well. Exercise? Maybe, but never enough. Friendships? Spirituality? Community? Who has the time? Or the inspiration? *The Big Question:* *"How about just surviving the day?"* Our lives are like a Quagmire, and it is often difficult to see beyond our muddy path.

Our lives are hectic. Most of us live in the day-to-day Quagmire, from morning to evening, absorbed in our unending schedules, commitments, errands, and responsibilities. The demands of life come at us hurriedly, piling more responsibilities on our bulging "to do" lists. We often have to schedule "me time" just to catch our breath. Even if we do take "me time," we spend it worrying about the things we are *not* doing.

If we barely have time for the basics of daily living, how then do we pay attention to our own well-being? Most of us don't, and significant parts of our lives begin to show signs of poor physical and emotional health through tight muscles, headaches, frequent colds, conflict in relationships, or problems on the job. Some people turn to alcohol or drugs; others experience anxiety or depression. In a spiraling fashion, signs of poor health aggravate the signs of distress. If we continue to lead our lives reactively in the fast-paced Quagmire of the twenty-first century, we will eventually find ourselves in crisis: a physical, mental, emotional, or spiritual breakdown.

Compounding this, the twenty-first century is considered a time for the proliferation of information that demands our attention. Our technological devices, computers, tablets, phones, television, and radios stream a blaring flow of data at us. We are bombarded daily with information about business, politics, and the world, about money, health, and sports, alongside hundreds of daily jokes and mottos for better living. News channels flood the airwaves with breaking news from around the world, opinions of "experts," points of view from complete strangers, and the thoughts of our friends on any topic that momentarily crosses their unique mindscape.

From the rampant flows of information and opinion, emotional sediment spreads across the consciousness of whole populations, countries and states, associations, groups of peers, and family members. We are constantly being influenced about what we should experience, think, and feel. Emotional influence drives much of our economy; it deeply affects our sense of global, national, and personal safety and motivates us into action.

With rapid two-way global interaction, information spreads within hours and minutes, public consciousness is influenced at will, and opinions spread across continents by the click of a cursor. Our own lives are impacted, our beliefs and values challenged by our time on the "net" informing us about who we should be and the world we live in. Our time in personal relationships is often interrupted by the constant chime of the cell phone or the call for electronic game-playing. Our personal oceans are roiling seas, with currents and undercurrents often in conflict and the threat of drowning always near.

Technology is a wonderful—terrible phenomenon. We can find and learn almost anything by searching the web and get it at the speed of light; we can talk to almost anyone about anything. But we can be constantly diverted away from our deeper selves. With the immediacy of our careers and our family responsibilities, we have scarce time for inner reflection, which means less time to really get to know ourselves and our families. Steady streams of news and world events constantly paint our inner environments dark as we are bombarded with a continuously fearful outlook on the world at large.

Further, we feel unsafe. On September 11, 2001, four airplanes were hijacked by terrorists: two were flown into the World Trade Center in New York City, one was flown into the Pentagon, and a fourth crashed in the Pennsylvania countryside. Thousands of lives were lost. It put a quick end to the sense of security in our country. Millions of people around the world watched the Twin Towers fall on television; news services ruthlessly streamed the incident at us and injected unprecedented fear and panic into our lives. Our relationship to safety for our families and communities changed in a single day, and we have never fully recovered. In fact, terrorist activities continue across the globe, changing the outlook of our lives, our political environment, and our personal safety within our own borders – and in our own hearts and minds.

What does life in the twenty-first century mean for our well-being, our physical health, and our sense of authentic spirituality? How do we firmly ground ourselves in the ever-changing Quagmire of our lives and live confidently into our finest inspirations? How does the Alchemist in us find the time to conduct our science?

Living into Our Core Beliefs

We spend every minute of every day living into our beliefs about who we are. That is how we maintain our grounding in the Quagmire. Like the waves of the sea, we trust in them, forming a consistent presence that will continue to brush the shores of our existence every day without exception. We know that our life experiences have ebb and flow, but we have confidence in the relative stability of those core beliefs about ourselves – they keep us grounded. If they ceased to exist for even a brief moment, we'd live in fear that our lives were in peril. That is how dearly we regard the core beliefs about ourselves and others.

So much do we trust our beliefs and the manner of the currents that ebb and flow in our lives, that every step we take, every action we conceive, is designed to prove their truth. This is what it is to "live into" a belief. It means that every step we take in life – and we take them only one at a time – is, moment by moment, designed to validate the truth of our beliefs. If we were to venture into another world of beliefs, we would feel adrift in unknown waters with no map to navigate, rudderless and without direction.

The majority of our core beliefs about ourselves are established in our first five years of life, those formative years when we form deep-seated conclusions about life and our own identity. Despite our deep-rooted feelings regarding our core beliefs, it is likely that only a fraction of them are true. Well-meaning (or not so well-meaning) adults and friends provide us, as we grow and mature, information about who we should be and what the experience of life is like. They inform us about who we are, how we should think and feel, and the type of people we should become.

The messages about our identities, the messages that form our core beliefs, rarely come to us in pure form. They can penetrate our consciousness directly, as in "You are such a loving child," or "Shame on you!" or they can come to us through the gesture of a smile or a scowl. A steady diet of simple inattention can signal abandonment and a sense of worthlessness to a child, and even the innocent (in) actions of perhaps well-meaning parents can inflict as much harm as physical abuse. Sometimes messages enter our consciousness two at time, as when a compliment is delivered through the eyes of jealousy. Psychologists call this a "double bind."

We, in our youthful innocence, take in all the messages and work out our own conclusions around conflicting evidence. We begin to form core beliefs about ourselves that allow us to survive; we mold our behaviors to please our parents or appease a punishment and conceive deep-seated theories about ourselves and the world. Those early formative experiences inform our core beliefs – our fundamental identities – and we spend most of our lives living into them, ensuring our survival.

My formative years taught me that my importance in the world was nearly nonexistent. Compared to the death of my father, not much mattered. My mother, largely living out her trauma, had little time for her own emotional repair, and as a result I believed that nothing short of my own death would result in receiving attention. Much of the time I felt invisible, unseen and unwitnessed. I held no worth. Invisibility, worthlessness, and being unseen extended beyond a few short experiences and became a core part of my bedrock beliefs. If my behavior drew attention, I promptly retreated into hiding to ensure my life was preserved according to belief.

I continued as the valiant girl living into my core belief of worthlessness, withdrawing when attention threatened to come my way, until one day a friend egged me on to buy a new lambskin-lined brown leather jacket. The guilt I felt from buying something luxurious for myself, especially something so extraordinarily exotic and costly, caused a deep panic that settled into my very center. Panic gave way to life-threatening terror, and I felt a clear and present sense that I was going to die. If my anxious tachycardia didn't kill me, something else was surely going to end me. I was experiencing a very steep undertow in the current of my psyche, and I was both startled and aghast, but yet intrigued that such an experience lived within me. I had crossed a boundary of a core belief about myself, and I was experiencing a strong physical reaction to it.

I kept the jacket – and I wore it. A part of me began to die that day: that part of my identity, my core belief that I was invisible and worthless. It was the first experience I had rocking the boat of my core belief system. It was not the last.

We live into our beliefs every day, a single step at a time as though we were clinging to a small buoy in a vast sea. Each step we take affirms the truth of our beliefs with the experience of peril like the sword of Damocles, threatening any deviation to the world as it should be.

As we learn the art of Alchemy, we begin to live an examined life – a masterful life – and we will learn to charter our territory, mix up the elements of our experience, and allow our natural inspiration to emerge. As a novice Alchemist, you will learn about the currents of your own life that dwell within, you will shoot the rapids and rest on the beaches of respite. You will learn the chemistry of your thoughts and feelings, perceive new vistas of experience, and gain the science, intuition, and knowledge to live a deeply inspired life.

I wholeheartedly encourage you to peek into your own *Book of Life Past* and see who you were and who you are now. I urge you to tease out, test, experiment, and challenge the core beliefs you are living into. Mix your feelings, your intelligence, and your experience with core beliefs...and, as did the Alchemists of old, you can create updated core beliefs, allowing fresh inspiration to flow freely!

I wish you Godspeed in exploring the dynamics of your internal currents and learning the art of your own personal alchemy. I rest on the sidelines of your adventure with eager anticipation, awaiting your discovery of the exhilaration of inspiration and the harnessing of its power. And finally, I wish you the grace of fortitude to explore your

Grand Mysteries, to ask the Big Questions, and to live with abandon into the Frontier Adventure of your inspired life.

Adventures in the Quagmire

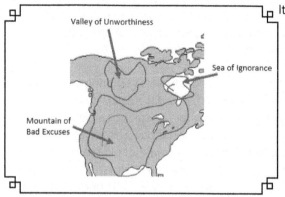

It's remarkable how resilient we are as humans. I have seen people of all ages weather childhood trauma, physical setbacks, devastating events in adolescence, and deep tragedy in adulthood. Many recover themselves with time, hard work, and the grace of spirit. Others aren't so fortunate, and they shiver down into unhappy shadows of their former selves. You need only observe a young toddler, unfettered by life's eventual mishaps, to get an idea of our human strength and vitality. We all have it in abundance. It may get bruised and abused throughout life's experience, but we have the built-in formidable ability, with effort, to regenerate. Innate to our marvelous human construction we have the great gifts of choice and fortitude, along with the biology of resilience. What an amazing adventure we can have as we enter the Quagmire of our daily lives!

Let's gear up to begin our adventure through the Quagmire, our daily experience where our busy, frenetic lives make the idea of living into inspiration sound like a pipe dream. Gearing up requires us to explore our overstimulated, under-examined, hurried lives and find a firm footing deeply rooted in strong, buoyant core beliefs. Once grounded, we are free to use our personal Alchemy to search for updated truths and release obsolete myths that no longer apply. Once we begin our journey, be assured that we will trek along many dark and muddy paths that can be scary at times, but gearing up properly will allow us the firm footing that prevents us from toppling. The pained and shadowy golems of our earlier life may dart out from the underbrush and block the path forward, but these are only shadows: flimsy, formless shapes that live beneath the binding of your *Book of Life Past*. Once exposed to the sunlight, they have no power, they bear no substance, and they become distant memories left behind in your chronicle of moments past. Cherish them, whatever their form, as they have become what Alchemists call the "base elements" of all that you are today.

The difficulty is that the obsolete core beliefs you bring to the trek through the Quagmire will make it difficult to successfully navigate. We may find ourselves in muddy waters or stuck in a blind valley that may hinder the journey forward for undue periods of time. As we adventure through the Quagmire, beware of old messages that hold no promise, slippery slopes where you keep falling down, and hidden traps that block your path. Should you find yourself stuck, this book should help you find some valuable grounding to help you gain powerful footholds and allow you safe passage through the territory. In this chapter, we find obstacles in the Quagmire that threaten your survival: Beware of 1) the Valley of Unworthiness (sense of self); 2) the Mountain of Bad Excuses (physical health); and 3) the Ocean of Despair (spirituality).

It is time to gear up! In the paragraphs that follow are some of the obsolete core beliefs you bring to the journey. Accompanying each of these are one or more footholds of truth (elements, to the Alchemist) to help you keep or regain your grounding. Grab on to the ones that fit and leave behind those that don't. It may be that be you have much different messages that follow you and cast shadows along your path. I encourage you to write them down, mark them up, comment in the margins, and expose them to the light of paper. See for yourself how the sunshine of perspective will lead you to firmer ground.

Grounding Your Sense of Self

Avoid the Valley of Unworthiness

At the start of our adventure we travel through a dry desert valley that spreads mounds of low shrubbery before us, a seeming wasteland where heatwaves radiating up from the ground create unusual mirages. These mirages reflect our sense of self, only the mirages sometimes appear ambiguous in appearance – some days looking safe and solid, while on others they look like ponds of rippling water. This is the Valley of Unworthiness, and it is known to change its appearance daily, depending on the messages that are blowing across the valley. We move in for closer inspection.

Our sense of self is the foundation, the very bedrock of who we know ourselves to be. Once we sort through our own messages about our sense of self, we can lay claim to our personal truths. Only when we see ourselves clearly can we then form clear perceptions of others. All of our perceptions color the world before us. If you see the world through angry or fearful shadows of the past, you have become lost in the Valley of Unworthiness, where you are destined for disappointment. Yet, if we spend the time to sift through and tease out our truths, we can draw forth our compassion as we remain firmly grounded to live into our inspiration.

Your Core Belief	New Grounding
Don't Be You	*Know Thyself*
One of the earliest challenges we face in life is the mandate to not be you. "Don't be angry," "Don't be sad," "Don't be selfish," "Don't be you." "Do be what others want you to be." Please your mother, obey your father, do as the teacher tells you, follow your boss, and please your spouse/partner. There is plenty of feedback that broadcasts the message that we are not doing things right – at least in the eyes of some others.	The ancient Greek maxim from the tenth century BC, "Know Thyself," is often offered up as guidance to pay no attention to the opinion of others over the truth of our own experience. No one can truly know what we perceive, what we want, why we do the things that we do better than ourselves. In our youth, inexperience fills us with self-doubt, but through trial and error, and through our deep sense of knowing, we come to learn who we are. Informed experience, deepened self-awareness, and intuitive knowing grow as we mature. They are elements for the Alchemist in you to use.

When you receive messages that you "can't be you," pause and remember the grounding of "Know thyself." Honor and trust your perceptions, your gut feelings. Align yourself with what you know to be true. As you honor your perceptions and gain confidence, you will become the best version of yourself with the information at hand. Be free to be you: play with your awareness, become sensitive to your gut feelings, test your instincts, and earn your own self-confidence. Take a firm stand in your own identity – challenge the core belief that "you can't be you" and *know* that "you can be you." |

Your Core Belief	New Grounding
You Are Not Worthy	*Esteem Yourself*

Expectations from others may diminish our innate capabilities or try to influence our decisions towards areas in which we hold no interest. At times, the expectations of others are colored by their own depleted self-esteem, or by shadowy images, yet they get projected onto us as the sound advice of an expert. Most have nothing to do with our own inner sense of direction and inevitably drag us down a false path or leave us feeling unworthy and "less than." Beware of the expectations of others for you, particularly those that deliver that deadly message: "You are not enough."

We must take it upon ourselves to acknowledge and value our "self," to give ourselves the esteem and the respect that nature intends for us. First, we must remember that maxim, "Know Thyself," and hold in high regard the strength and value we bring to situations both small and large. For example, if you know yourself to be a level-headed person, value that aspect of yourself and know you bring level-headed, considered thinking to a situation. If you are a creative soul, value the creativity you bring into the world, your out-of-the-box thinking, or the sense of beauty and art that you offer to those around you. This is self-esteem, the deep respect and value we hold toward our unique talents and strengths. These are the attributes of grace and well-being that recognize our fullness and honor our strengths, the gifts we bring into the lives of others – the tools we use to make a better world for our family, our friends and our communities.

Esteem Others

We must be able to hold ourselves in high esteem before we can esteem others. Valuing self and others is the basis, the very foundation of solid relationship. Focusing on the weaknesses of ourselves and others does nothing more than add "just another brick in the wall" of a self-imposed barrier. Esteem yourself, hold others in high regard, and build relationship foundations that support growth and vitality. Bring forth the best in yourself and in others.

Your Core Belief	New Grounding
Don't Speak Your Truth	*Stop, Look, and Listen*
One lifelong challenge in our relationships is learning how to identify problems and concerns, and then articulating and communicating constructively about them. Hurt feelings, anger, frustration, and fear motivate the worst behaviors in all of us. We say and do hurtful things, we push people away and others do the same with us. Feelings, emotions, and hurtful behaviors are simply *indicators* that let us know that we need something that we are not getting. Period. No blame, no attribution: just something missing in our own experience. Yet we fear gently speaking our deepest truth from the grounding of our own esteem. Reacting in the heat of the moment doesn't work to our advantage; in fact, it tends to increase the problem's intensity and leave us far less informed than we were initially.	When difficult situations arise, "Stop, Look, and Listen." We must be able to identify harmful behaviors by looking at all sides of a situation and listening to our conscious awareness for what might be missing in our experience. Listen to the voice deep within for self-understanding, for perspective, and for your own permission to want what you want, to need what you need, and to think what you think. Create quiet space and listen to the whisperings of your heart; then, and only then, speak the truth about what you need.
	You Are Always Communicating
	We are *always* communicating. What we don't communicate in some way out into the world will express itself, disguised in our body language and our behavior. As we begin to ground ourselves in our own truth, deepen our sense of esteem, and honor the events of our lives, we come to understand that we are always communicating. The avoidance of outward communication is often expressed internally in the form of stress-related symptoms or even illness. Honor your wellness and your relationships by speaking your truth. Be fully you.
	Our lives matter to us and to those around us: our spouses, parents, children, coworkers, and friends. Do your communications add value to the situation at hand, or do you create "drag" and resistance to clarity and progress, to health and growth? You are always communicating: speak your truth with discernment and kindness, since you are the creator and ultimate recipient of your own well-being.

Your Core Belief	New Grounding
Wait and Follow	*Leadership Is an Imperative*
How many times have you taken the initiative in your life, only to be told by a boss, spouse, or friend that you chose improperly? Perhaps your choices interrupted someone's agenda, or breached another's core beliefs. Who knows, but the message is clear that you should follow their lead, abandon what you know, and follow in their footsteps. This begs the question of possible gaps in perception, conflicting directions, and/or leadership in your own life.	How many people do not overcome the challenge of leadership and pass the baton of vitality on to other people in their lives? We cannot hide behind the veneer of meekness, indecision, or passivity if we are to fully live into our inspiration and claim ownership of our contributions in this world. Who have you chosen to become? The passive recipient of bad luck, bad genes, bad choices...? Or have you chosen the path of personal leadership – choosing to live into your inspiration, expanding your life according to your own pace, and, by virtue of the nature you were given, providing contributions to your family, friends, and community?
	Know When to Surrender
	There are times when leadership in your life's contributions are an imperative, but there are also times to surrender to those things that you cannot or should not change. It is important to understand those things that you cannot change, like someone else's point of view – they are not yours to change. There will always be roadblocks on your path, some you can do something about and others that are immovable. It is important to recognize the difference and embrace surrender.
	Leadership, surrender, and the wisdom to choose between these are the hallmarks of balanced living. Taking your place in relationships, valuing your contributions, and living into your inspiration give all parties the calm, serenity, and safety absolutely needed to fulfill each person's potential.

Grounding Your Physical Health

Don't Get Sidetracked on the Mountain of Bad Excuses

As we traverse the Quagmire and gain a firmer grounding in our sense of self, we will encounter a majestic, forested mountain of spreading oaks, granite walls, and slimy parasites nesting in moist crevasses. It teems with life. Our own physical health is what provides us with the stamina, strength, and endurance to navigate each day with ease and comfort, allowing us to gain confidence and satisfaction. Our bodies need sufficient energy to sustain the requirements of daily living and enough energy to work, raise a family, and enjoy our lives. We also need to have sufficient endurance and resilience to restore our energy and recover from physical and emotional stress and mental fatigue. We all know this, but it's so tempting to take inviting shortcuts on paths that appear easier than the planned ascent. During our trek over the Mountain of Bad Excuses, we get waylaid as apparent shortcuts lead us back to the base of the trail, where we must begin again. Bad Excuses are everywhere and are fully supported by cultural norms, demanding jobs, and the fast food industry. Like a parasite, they feed off our poor sense of self and seek out the tired and vulnerable. As we gear up for our twenty-first-century adventure, we must study the map so we can identify and avoid inviting shortcuts. Take a look at the slippery slopes below and equip yourself with vigilance and stable boundaries that will enable you to retain firm grounding through the ups and downs of the Quagmire.

No matter how prepared we think we are, we undoubtedly will still lose our balance from time to time and fall backwards as we make our ascent. What is it that causes us to lose our grounding and allows us to slip back into the muck? A large area of the Quagmire is mountainous; it is a challenging experience and difficult to traverse. Our lack of attention to our physical health affects people throughout the world. The influence of our cultural norms and the economic climate has become a concern of national and global proportions.

34

In our own lives, we fall out of balance as we spend so much of our time reactively meeting the demands of our jobs, families, and other commitments over the needs of our own well-being. It may feel like we have no choice, but we absolutely do. In fact, it's all about choice.

As we venture through our experience on the Mountain of Bad Excuses and feel the draw of the shortcuts with slippery slopes, gear up with the following to hold your ground.

Slippery Slope	Grounding
Wellness as An Aspiration It is all too easy to hold wellness as an aspiration for the future. Sure, we feel good now, so we tell ourselves, "I can put on my coat of better habits tomorrow." But the mysterious nature of time keeps us forever in "the now," with "tomorrow's" arrival only a mental marker that never arrives. This slippery slope of time is dangerous, yet elusive, as our innocuous choices in the present moment become deeply embedded habits. They quietly gather momentum in our bodies and minds, until eventual physical, mental, or even spiritual crisis erupts. Are you living into wellness, or awaiting the adventure of catastrophe?	*Live into Wellness* We live our lives through the choices we make every moment of every day, and we journey through life one step at a time, one choice at a time. Choose to live into wellness: it is not an aspiration! It is a here-and-now state of consciousness. You are sifting through your mysteries, asking big questions, and making choices as you read this paragraph. You either choose to live into wellness, or you don't. Hungry? Do you choose to eat an apple or a bag of chips? Overweight? Is it TV or a nice walk? Finally, if you choose to live into wellness, claim it as your choice. If you choose to live into eventual catastrophe, then claim that as your choice. Be honest: the only person you can fool is yourself – just ask the onlookers of your journey. *Tell Yourself the Truth* Most of us consider ourselves to be basically honest people, right? Then why do we lie to ourselves about our wellness and our bodies? Why do we doggedly defend ourselves against our own truth? I marvel at the technology that allows us to track our calories, our heart rates, and activity levels, and then share our readings with our online friends. I marvel even more at the lies we tell ourselves that become shared information. I watched my husband once consume a bowl of nuts, yet in his calorie counter he recorded "1 ounce, mixed nuts." Really? Embrace your truths and lay claim to your choices; uncover your mysteries, great and small. Beg the big questions and allow your answers to emerge. Only then can you live into your wellness.

Slippery Slope	Grounding
Selective Amnesia	*Value Wellness*
It can be difficult to place value on something that you already have. A fish doesn't really value water until it is placed on a dry surface. If you have experienced a health crisis in your past you likely place a higher value on wellness than do the uninitiated. But even if your wellness becomes stable, you are always on the fertile ground of selective amnesia. This quicksand in the Quagmire sucks you in slowly and is deceptively difficult to get out of. The phrase "time heals" is a sound maxim, but as time passes, the original event becomes only a chapter in your chronicle of life past and becomes buried in your memory.	Stand quietly outside and gaze at the nature that surrounds you. The world is aglow with vibrant plants reaching to the skies; perhaps a distant horizon traces the cool outlines of hills or the silhouettes of buildings once fresh and newly painted. Perhaps the landscape is peppered here and there with long ignored, starving growth or with buildings aged into artifacts bereft of their original intent. Self-neglect, or selective amnesia, only pulls you back into the original sinkhole, as old habits reemerge and recreate the problems you first experienced.

Once you recover the wellness you once had lost and selective amnesia begins to settle into your heart and mind, continue the practices you began in the heat of panic. Let them become rituals that you perform and bring to them your resistance; resist your desires to slip back into old habit. Resistance itself is a mystery, the reemergence of older shadows. Chase down the big questions; sit in stillness and allow your inspiration to drive. As a novice Alchemist, you may wrestle with the practice, but as your mastery grows, your inspiration will emerge and naturally call you into the heart of well-being. |

Slippery Slope	Grounding
Locus of Control We often use defensive techniques to reassure ourselves that maintaining our wellness is really out of our control. The popular shortcut of "Out of My Hands" is a warehouse of entertaining excuses: "I don't have time to cook," "I don't have time to exercise," "I'm out of shape," "I'm too old," "I'm not old enough," "It's not my fault." Yet somehow we can carve out time to talk with a friend on the phone or chat with coworker in the office, or, better yet, find some unwitting bystander to blame. The desire to blame is based on what is called in psychology "an external locus of control," where we believe that outside events or people are responsible for the misfortunes in our lives.	*You Are the Creator of Your Own Life* This may sound like a harsh and heavy cross to bear, but in reality, it is the core belief that brings to you vast vistas of freedom. Years ago, I was assigned a job well below my professional level and expertise. I blamed a bad boss, performance misperceptions, and a host of other potential targets. Then, in one of those quiet, reflective moments I begged the Big Question: "How did I attract this situation? Me, the owner of this awful experience." The answer came in an instant as I acknowledged the degree to which I had been under intense stress for the last several years. My inner knowing quickly provided a very poignant, yet simple response: "You are tired; take this time to recover." We tend to look outside of ourselves for answers and actually seek out shortcuts, yet the truth lives within the deeper currents of our lives. We have the answers: we just need to beg the questions and then await our own voice of wisdom, the voice of our inner truths that already knows and is awaiting your question.

Grounding Your Spirituality

Walk Away from Ignorance

Spirituality in the twenty-first century appears to be a shifting phenomenon. In the early to mid-1900s, spirituality was usually aligned with an organized religion. If you asked someone if they were spiritual, they would generally say they were Jewish, Catholic, Protestant, Muslim, Buddhist, Hindu, and so on. Some might align with a religion – say, Judaism – but claim to be an agnostic or an atheist, while others might say they were not religious at all. Spirituality was primarily linked to some form of religious affiliation.

Around the 1970s, as New Age thinking began to emerge, people began to classify their spirituality apart from traditional religious affiliation. A standalone sense of spirituality appealed to those unfulfilled by traditional religious practices. New-Agers gained a refreshed sense spiritual freedom, unhindered by restrictive and dated rituals.

Religious persecution and annihilation have plagued humanity throughout our entire history. The fear of discrimination, confinement, or death has left us with thousands of years of deep scar tissue. If you are in a group of people very different from yourself you may feel the need to hide your true identity, lest you experience rejection, discrimination, or something far worse. This is the Sea of Difference, and it has harmed millions of disenfranchised souls. You may brush up against the riptides of difference in unfamiliar social gatherings or experience it at a political rally. It is experienced as the need to remain silent as peril is in your presence. *Do not* allow yourself to be drawn in or trapped by it: the preservation of your very spirit depends upon your spiritual freedom.

The truth is that we have highly sensitive perceptive radar, and by sending out and receiving radar signals we can be warned about this trap in the Quagmire – ignorance.

Trap	Self-Preservation Strategy
Ignorance	*Walk Away from Ignorance*
Simply put, ignorance and the lack of sensitivity and awareness is at the root of discrimination. So many situations in our lives deliver some very Grand Mysteries. In research conducted by psychologist Albert Ellis in the 1950s, looking at discrimination shown in the Holocaust and other historical events, it was concluded that we fear people that are not like ourselves and that these fears are transmitted intra-generationally.	Cultivate sensitivity and awareness. Be aware that the fear of differences is a deeply ingrained set of core beliefs and is not readily available for influence. Rather than poke at the edges of ignorance, steer clear and pursue the life that inspires you. That is your path, the Way of your life. It's the only way.
	Value Your Sense of Spirituality
On a small scale, discrimination arises every day as we meet people with very different opinions or points of view. There is a lot we can learn a lot about the nature of man and our own spirit; however, for those unwilling to ask Big Questions and listen to their deep inner guidance, ignorance remains firmly entrenched.	Go back to the earlier section on Sense of Self and reread it again and again. Don't be distracted by the ignorance of others. It's a false path: it only impedes your own journey and sucks you down into the Sea of Differences.

Through the Eyes of Youth

Always know that you are perfect just as you are, and that all the bumps and bruises you have collected thus far in your life are hard-earned adventure badges from life in the Quagmire. But when do we actually stop and notice that our horribly dated core beliefs and lifestyles are causing us harm? Perhaps the trigger is a diagnosis of diabetes or high blood pressure, or perhaps a relationship that is in troubled waters. At some point events in our lives *will* give us a firm message to stop, take a good look at ourselves, and find a better way.

We have been gifted remarkably resilient bodies, filled with the sensitive perceptive instruments of our senses, amazingly sharp intellects, and the deep desire to ignite body, mind, and spirit in pursuit of the lives that we yearn for. The earlier we listen to the warning signs in our lives, the easier it will be to return not only to a state of well-being, but to venture forward as the incredible power of our free-flowing inspiration fuels our journey in remarkable new directions.

Learning the Alchemy of experience requires a deeper understanding, a new framework through which to view our internal and external environments...how their dynamics subtly shape our experience and how we can skillfully navigate them with clarity of perspective, stable core beliefs, and a detailed map of the territory.

With this book you can pause and find respite as we gear ourselves up for our Frontier Adventure. You may sometimes glance back through the scrapbook of your *Book of Life Past* for memorable pearls of wisdom, or prepare for today's adventures using the skills of the Alchemist. You will find many Great Mysteries in the Quagmire of your life and ask the Big Questions. I promise you that their answers are quite simple and will offer you sweet relief.

Experiment viewing your life from the Alchemist's perspective, embrace your Frontier Adventure in the Quagmire, and experience it through the youthful eyes of delight and intrigue that remain intact deep within. Each frayed parchment page of your *Book of Life Past* will become a treasure-trove of life's singular moments. Good and bad alike, they shaped you into the miracle you are today.

If you experience trepidation or pause, remember that childhood holds only the flimsy shadows of another time, which drizzle and dissolve as they become exposed to the light of today. Look for the messages, slippery slopes, and traps of belief and apply the firm groundings from this chapter as you proceed forward along your path.

As you become the Alchemist of your own experience, you will learn to master the powerful currents that ebb and flow within and around you. You will be able to create for yourself a safe space for rest and respite that will allow your inspiration the freedom to flow freely, a space that will help your yearnings crystallize and power your energies to create the life you desire.

~

Once again, you quietly drift into your earlier reverie of your own *Book of Life Past* as it lies before you. Its soft leather binding begs for your attention, as you trace your delicately engraved name on its worn leather cover and run your fingers over the embossed image of the dancer. Somehow you know it is now up to you to conceive your future, to learn how to live into the life that inspires you. As you embark on your journey seeking your Grand Mystery, you know that you are returning to the life that calls to you from some long-forgotten daydream.

CORE BELIEFS SUMMARIZED

GROUNDING THE SELF

- ➢ You are perfect – right now
- ➢ Be strong, know thyself
- ➢ Honor your strengths, and hold yourself in high esteem
- ➢ Honor others with clear-sighted esteem

- ➤ Stop, look, and listen; then speak your truth

- ➤ Know that you are always communicating

- ➤ Personal leadership is an imperative; take your own initiative

- ➤ Surrender to the things that you cannot change; do it quickly

GROUNDING YOUR PHYSICAL HEALTH

- ➤ Live into Wellness – moment by moment

- ➤ Keep your truths visible

- ➤ *You* are the creator of your own well-being

GROUNDING YOUR SPIRITUALITY

- ➤ Walk away from ignorance

- ➤ Value your spiritual sense of self; avoid distractions

Alchemist's Practice

A Page from Your Book of Life Past

1. Think about a period in your life that you would like to explore and spend about 30–60 minutes writing a Chronicle about it. You might describe the events or experiences of that period and reflect on any portion of it you wish to explore.

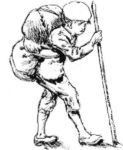

There are no rules, no boundaries, and no wrong approaches. Simply allow yourself free rein to express yourself.

Take a break and come back later to Alchemist's Practice Step 2 with a refreshed mind.

2. Reread the Chronicle you wrote in Step 1 and pick out all the messages, slippery slopes, and traps you can find. See if you can infer additional messages in your chronicle as you read between the lines. List them below. Alongside each obstacle you identify, write an updated alternative that will help you stay grounded:

Sense of Self

Obsolete Messages   Updated Messages

_____   _____

_____   _____

_____   _____

_____   _____

Physical Health

Slippery Slopes   New Practice

_____   _____

_____   _____

_____   _____

_____   _____

Spirituality

Traps of Ignorance   Strategy

_____   _____

_____   _____

_____   _____

_____   _____

3. As you sift through your core beliefs, do any Great Mysteries or Big Questions arise? List them below:

Great Mysteries   Big Questions

_____   _____

_____   _____

_____   _____

_____   _____

4. What was your experience completing this activity?

∞

Chapter 2

~

Living into Wellness

"All of life is an evolving Grand Mystery, so do what inspires you and be well enough to do it."

~

Find it yourself, Its inside and out,
It has no beginning You have it No doubt.

—J. K. S. Zetlan

"My reveries seem to come and go!" you lament as you ground your thumbs in to your aching temples. "I have almost forgotten how to dream, and anyway, I have no energy for aging fantasies. I wouldn't even know where to begin!"

~

To enable us to live into inspiration, we must be well enough for the journey. We don't need to have *perfect* Wellness for our inspiration to flourish, but it is important to have a sense of well-being, a feeling of satisfaction that we are moving in the right direction – if for no other reason than to know that we are making steady progress.

In any journey, we all experience peaks and valleys, and none will be more difficult, or exhilarating, than navigating the path that enables you to live into inspiration. Perhaps, as you start your own journey, you worry that the path is steep and that you are out of shape. The place to begin the journey, then, is by focusing on your Wellness today.

Wellness is a Grand Mystery in its own right, and all who live in the Quagmire know of its quest. Many people think that they have found Wellness, but most would be unable to tell you exactly how they found it...and even fewer would be prepared to tell you how they *created* it. The quest for Wellness begs the singularly Big Question: "What is it?" directly followed by the quest of, "How do I get to it?" The answers are simple; the journey is challenging.

In my personal quest for Wellness, I encountered many obstacles. As an example, about the time I edged over from young adulthood to middle age I became very ill. In one year I counted the onset of thirty-two different viruses making me very sick and unusually fatigued. This lasted for over three years without a single day of feeling well. I had been married less than a year and had recently given birth to a beautiful son. My job, over an hour's commute away, was part of my dream career, yet each morning when I woke up I thought perhaps I should have been hospitalized.

I visited many specialists over the course of those three years, but no single professional was able to put a finger on the illness. I visited internists, specialists in communicable diseases, psychologists, nutrition specialists, chiropractors, and energy workers. None had the solution, although each one tried to treat me with their medicine of choice – to no avail.

> *"[High Level Wellness is] an integrated method of functioning which is oriented toward maximizing the potential of which the individual is capable. It requires that the individual maintain a continuum of balance and purposeful direction within the environment where he is functioning. "*
>
> *–Halbert L. Dunn, MD, circa 1956*

But as a wife and a new mother with a career I was happy...yet depressed; deeply connected with the beauty of my life...but too physically sick to enjoy it. Despite constantly pushing myself forward, I was torn – wanting to be a good wife, but falling short; a good mother, but too exhausted; and an aggressive business woman, but feeling too ill to impress anyone with my talent.

In my deepest heart I wanted to be "normal" but felt clueless on how to achieve it. Wellness became a burning Grand Mystery of my middle years, and I began a quest for it that continues to this day. Through this experience and that of others, I learned a lot about the way towards wellness and now enjoy many rewards resulting from that difficult journey.

> *Wel-nis: "The general state of well-being, generally associated with the presence of human emotions possessing generally happy, optimistic qualities ..."* also:
>
> *"...The slowest possible rate at which one can die."*
>
> –Urban Dictionary

Wellness often feels elusive. In fact, the concept of wellness has only been around since the mid-1950s and was brought to the forefront of medicine by Halbert L. Dunn, MD in the context of alternative medicine. Before the '50s, people were considered healthy – or not – depending simply on the presence or absence of illness or disease. It was a narrow definition, with other areas of the whole person segmented into mental health or religion. For example, if you were physically healthy but suffered from depression, you were still well; if you suffered from stress-related headaches, you had a medical problem and got treated with painkillers. The world has come a long way since the 1950s, in terms of better understanding wellness as a question of the whole person. However, the definition of wellness is still undergoing significant changes.

In a series of lectures at the Unitarian Universalist Church in Arlington, Virginia (circa 1956), Dunn introduced the phrase "high level wellness" and reframed the concept of "wellness" into one that encompasses a far broader experience than merely the presence or absence of disease. He brought into the conversation the integrated roles of body, mind, spirit, *and* environment as being instrumental in reaching our individual human potential.

In the modern world that brings us pesticides, air pollution, non-essential medications, and an ever-growing list of toxins and other contaminants, we cannot dismiss the profound impact that our external environment has upon our internal environment – our wellness. Architects and landscapers are quick to acknowledge the impact the environment has on our individual states of mind. Psychologists have long recognized the powerful impact of these emotional states on our physical wellness.

Therefore, as we journey towards Wellness, we must recognize that our environments, both internal and external, are significant contributors to our wellness.

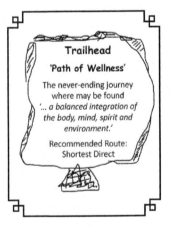

We are coming to understand an even richer meaning to the concept of wellness. The Urban Dictionary, a common-usage online dictionary of everyday language, has built a bridge from Wellness as observable science into the subjective realms of consciousness and emotion. As humans, we continue to chart a deeper course into understanding wellness with the proposition that achieving it will result not only in a longer life, but a life that also is more meaningful and emotionally satisfying.

As we begin our adventure through life's Quagmire of challenges, we enter the trailhead to the Path of Wellness.

To live into wellness and explore our Grand Mysteries, we must keep ourselves fit for the journey. In this section, we are going to explore wellness from four different perspectives: body, mind, spirit, and environment. We will explore those individual aspects of ourselves in turn, to better understand them individually. Later, in Part II, we will learn to recombine them with finesse, loving-kindness, and ease. When we understand these each in their own right, it is much easier to see a problem or challenge and self-correct, or even add something new to the mix.

Aspects of Ourselves / Holistic Wellness

How often do we stop and think about what Wellness is?

Most of the time we see ourselves as the holistic "I": "I am happy," "I am tired," or "I am a role (husband/wife/accountant/etc.)." We also know that we have different aspects of ourselves that make up the "Me"; we have our bodies, our minds, and our spirits. We move about in a number of different environments including our homes, cars, workplaces, cities, etc.

Wellness of Body

Our bodies are our physical resource for moving about in our environment. We depend on them to get from one place to another; to work, to raise our children, to be with those that we cherish, and even to love. Our bodies help determine the comfort of our ride through the Quagmire as we seek out our Big Mysteries.

As we gaze in the Lake of Reflection we see ourselves, and know that we are made of bones, muscles, tendons, and ligaments, each of which offer a wondrous concoction of physical "stuff" that holds us all together. Our bodies, sewn together by bones and connective tissues, house our organs, alongside our nervous and respiratory systems. Our blood transports oxygen and vital nutrients throughout our body through vast networks of arteries and veins. Our lymphatic system distributes hormones throughout our bodies, regulating our body systems and even allowing us to reproduce ourselves through the miracle of children. Through our skin, ears, nose, and eyes we receive our environment's vibration and translate the data into something meaningful. But as we gaze in the mirror of the lake, we see only our body – the shape of ourselves – our physical flaws.

While we often focus on our physical body we generally pay little attention to our bodies as a distinct part of a larger self, the total "me." When we wake up in the morning, "*we*" get up and begin our daily routine. *"We"* may lie in bed for a few minutes, lost in thought about the day to come, and then roll ourselves out of bed when we feel ready. Some of us feel that early-morning energy surge, while some are a part of the groggy millions awaiting their first cup of coffee. Some of us experience stiffness or limited flexibility after waking. All of us start the day differently, but as we arise to the day, we become more aware of that part of us that is our body.

Many of us are good at listening to our bodies – to know when we are well or if something is amiss. Sometimes, though, we are so entwined with our emotions and mental ruminations that we cannot hear the messages our bodies are sending to us. We stop listening.

A few years ago, I was working in downtown Oakland and commuting over an hour each way to work and back. One day I noticed I had become unusually cranky and had no patience to deal with my coworkers. I was short with them and was feeling terribly stressed out. I was having difficulty with my boss at the time: speaking with him was like rubbing sandpaper on a wound. Instead of relaxing over a nice dinner with my husband, I found him in a bad mood as well. I sought a bit of solitude in our living room. I lay on the couch, curled up in a little ball, and just let my mind wander. I was hoping to get to the bottom of whatever emotional problems were nipping at my mood and to resolve them as quickly as possible.

After about ten minutes of curling up in silence, words began to form on each of my exhales. I would inhale, and then breathe out the words, "Too much stress," or, "Let me be," or, "Just go away." With each exhale, I seemed to come deeper into my physical self. One by one, each exhale let out a phrase of exhaustion as I began to center more deeply within the quiet of my body. I wasn't trying to think about anything; the words just came as much-needed utterances. Not long after I began to exhale my body's cries of exhaustion, I began to notice that my stomach was upset and my chest and my lungs felt heavy. Under all the thoughts of irritation, frustration, and anger at everyone around me, I began to notice that I was sick.

Indeed, I had the flu. I felt horrible; however, I was so wound up in my thoughts, the daily routine of commuting, and spending so much of my time in meetings and discussions with other people that I had lost connection with my body. I was so used to being immersed in thought and emotion and the act of problem solving that I had neglected to listen to my body's language. I was deaf to its communications that were telling me, "You are ill."

It is easy to overlook our physical bodies, especially when we feel well. When we feel well, we have energy; we are eager to move about, and our moods are generally good. Unless we bump up against some form of physical limitation, we tend to ignore the language of our bodies. But we miss so much by turning a deaf ear to physical experience.

Positive experiences send our bodies messages as well. Have you ever gone outside the day after a rain and noticed the clear, crisp, cool air as it rests on your face and spontaneously thought, "This feels good," as you breathed in the freshly cleansed air? There's even a special word for this delicate after-rain smell: "petrichor." Perhaps the feel of the sun on your skin and the renewed sense of clarity on the horizon make you feel light. Who would want to miss such a moment, when the earth speaks so directly to our bodies and our bodies delight so intimately with the experience?

The body has a language of its own. It feels, sees, hears, and touches the world around us, and it always responds with what I call *native feelings and thoughts*. Native feelings and thoughts are those experiences that occur in the *here and now* – but then recede as quickly as they arose. In the receptive mode of pure experience, the deep connection to our senses comes alive; we become aware of our native feelings and thoughts as they spontaneously arise – *before* our preconditioned mind assigns them lengthier dialogue or more complicated feelings.

As with the experience of the clear day after a rain, as we soak in the sunshine and bask in its pleasure, we revel in the clarity of experience – these are native feelings and native thoughts. This is life in its simplest and *most complete* form – the language of our body.

There are multitudes of articles on health and wellness accessible to us, as well as many professionals who can examine, diagnose, and treat signs of ill health. However, my perspective is that we have abundant knowledge about the wellness of our bodies at all times – and that if we stay *tuned in* to our native feelings and thoughts we will know when we are off balance or have a problem. I am in no way suggesting we diagnose ourselves if we don't feel well, or that we discount the importance of medical examination and treatment. Our advances in medicine and alternative wellness are quite impressive. *I am, however, suggesting we become better listeners to the language of our bodies.*

Life in the Quagmire is intense. We get so busy that we forget to stop and listen to our bodies and take in the world that surrounds us. We get so absorbed in our emotions, recycled thinking, and stressful commitments that we just chug through the day to get things done. But when we forget to listen to the language of our body, we set ourselves up to miss early warning signs of stress or illness, or, alternatively, perhaps we miss the opportunity to experience the vibration of excitement or the warmth of contentment. In either case, we miss out on vital information.

Describing physical wellness, then, from the Alchemist's perspective, we are looking at how closely we are listening to the language of the body, the language of our native thoughts and feelings, and responding with compassion and responsibility. If we are inattentive to what our body is feeling, or how we are natively responding to our experience, the Alchemist would say we are putting ourselves at risk of illness or dysfunction. Although you may not be exhibiting signs of sickness at the moment, you are likely turning a deaf ear on the early warning signs of encroaching physical strain or breakdown.

People who practice yoga become keenly aware of their physical bodies and native experience. Getting into yoga postures takes a great deal of awareness about where your body parts are, how you are using them, and how pleasant the experience is. Yoga instructors generally give physical cues such as "Draw your shoulders away from your ears," "Gather the muscles on your back," or "Internally rotate your inner thighs." They might also suggest, "Find your edge," meaning that you should attend to how your body is feeling in the moment, respect your immediate physical limits, and don't push to extend beyond what feels good.

Yogis learn to look within physically and attend to their native feelings and thoughts as part and parcel of their practice. As a result, they gain tremendous insight into the physical well-being within their skin, moment by moment. Off the mat, yoga practitioners become incredibly adept at identifying physical problems before they become pronounced and can often shift their behavior on a dime to correct a problem.

You don't need to do yoga to develop internal physical awareness and become aware of native feelings and thoughts: it simply takes paying close attention to how your body is feeling and listening to its voice – something we in our culture are trained to ignore or even override.

If we are not used to tuning into our bodies, the experience can feel a bit scary and unnerving. It does take courage and self-compassion to allow native feelings and thoughts to arise. But to experience greater physical wellness, it is imperative that we start by meeting the world where we are – courageously – and to honor our body's native feelings and thoughts. Listen with a gentle and forgiving heart and know that you have come a very long way on the journey of your one precious life. Take the time to experience the body you came in on!

As you practice the art of listening to the language of your body, steer your life ever closer to those things that make you feel good; walk away from painful native experience. As we listen to the language of our bodies and respond to them respectfully, they will *never* lead us astray. Our bodies, our miles of interconnected "stuff," are our most informative resource on the planet and the greatest Frontier Adventure navigation device we will ever encounter. Try not to be led astray by random thoughts and emotions. *Instead, focus on listening to your body.*

Clarity of Mind

The mind, chief navigator of our journey, gives us an ongoing stream of information about our trek through the Quagmire. Our very wellness depends on our clarity of mind to process our experience, draw conclusions, and make important, life-sustaining decisions. It is a marvel of non-physical activity and bristling energy that guides our lives and creates our future!

Although we can speak about the mind and scientifically study the brain's composition, no one can assuredly tell us what it is. We can all attest to the fact that from the time we wake up in the morning until the time we go to sleep at night, we run an incessant internal dialogue complete with thoughts, plans, observations, stories, feelings, hunches, intuitions, and more. Even as we sleep, we can be deep in thought, as we experience dreams that are often full of vivid adventure and imagery, unusual characters with surprising conversations, and uncensored feelings and emotions.

What's inside our invisible mental containers? Our minds are a jumble of truths, fictions, wild and stored-up emotions, knowledge, and changing ideas. To successfully navigate the path to wellness, our job is to learn to uncover the mind's patterns, master its challenges, refine our skills, and allow our minds to do their real work – to inform us, with clarity, about the world. But to do that, we must first understand how the mind works.

In Buddhist philosophy, the mind has no physical shape, no color, no content, no texture, and no location, yet it plays perceptions across our "mindscape" and cognizes, or processes, our native experience. As we gather information through living, we begin to name, sort, classify, and otherwise sift through information as we need it. Mind is always aware of the content of our experience; it is that part of us that processes our experience.

Our closest and most intimate experience of the world is through our perceptions – the native experience of our bodies, feelings and thoughts. Following immediately on the heels of our experience, however, our minds begin to process the information and interpret their meaning which becomes our "personal truth." These are secondhand experiences, or manufactured byproducts, of our original experience: emotion and thought. Our personal truths are often accurate reflections of what we have experienced. However, sometimes we encounter a difficulty in our processing, where we make incorrect associations between our native experiences and draw flawed interpretations. This is the experience of The Bog, where the adventurer must learn of its many distractions and blind alleys and learn to cut a clear path through its troubled logic.

In a freshman psychology course in college I learned of a landmark study done in the early 1920s by two behavioral scientists, Watson and Rayner. They showed a soft and tame rabbit to Little Albert, a nine-month-old infant. Little Albert showed no fear of the animal and was quite comfortable near it, even reaching a hand out to touch its soft fluffy coat. Little Albert encountered the soft animal with calm and curiosity – what we might consider his natural experience of native feeling and thought.

As part of the study, however, the researchers placed Little Albert on the floor, then, shortly after seeing the rabbit, made a very loud and unpleasant noise behind the child, frightening him. The sound of the noise *paired* with the presence of the rabbit was repeated once a week for seven weeks. After the initial trials, when Little Albert was placed on the floor with the rabbit he would cry, show signs of distress, and try to crawl away. His initial calm and curiosity, his native feelings, had been buried beneath this new fear, a *paired* feeling, that was not directly related to the rabbit, but which occurred, nonetheless, very close in time. The initial experience paired with the loud noise produced a *new association* – rabbit and fear – that overrode Little Albert's native feeling. This is *emotion; a manufactured feeling that is the result of illogically paired experience.*

Unfortunately, the pairing of a soft white rabbit with a frightening noise produced such an intense reaction in Little Albert that he began to generalize his fear to other objects that resembled the rabbit, such as fluffy cotton fabric, a fur coat, and other similar items. Like Little Albert, we are often not aware of such conditioning in our own lives, but it happens all the time. We build up layers of paired emotion and thoughts; inadvertent events layered upon native experience. Then we act on our manufactured emotions as if they were real.

When I was younger, I had an easy and immediate trust with people: I simply knew people were honest. I always had some measure of pleasant experience with everyone, friend or otherwise, and had no reason to assume otherwise. Some people I liked, others not so much, but I had no reason to distrust anyone. I eventually met and married a lovely man who promised me what all young women wanted at the time – a chance to live the American Dream with a caring spouse, a roof over my head and, a beautiful child. To me, I had it all. There was no greater joy than coming home after a day's work, seeing the faces of my husband and curly-haired son, and spending long, pleasant evenings with them. Things weren't always perfect, as they never are in real life, but we always managed to talk and compromise through our differences. Some difficulties were harder than others, but I loved and trusted this man with my life, with my son, with my heart.

On what I now call "That Dark Day in August," my husband and I had a disagreement about what to do on his upcoming birthday. I had spent months training for a long-distance run and did not want to compromise my hoped-for performance by staying out late the night before the big race. A discussion about the birthday evening turned into a disagreement that escalated into a terrible physical assault. For no clear reason, I was beaten severely about the head and chest and left stranded on our front lawn in the chilly August night without my wits about me and without a husband. End of marriage.

As the days passed, I tried desperately to make sense out of what happened. Not just the disagreement, but the abrupt turnabout of reality: love to hurt, discussion to violence, fun to dissolution. Where did this violent behavior come from? How could I not see what was coming? Even after the physical pain of the native experience had long vanished, and after repeatedly playing out the experience in my mind to try to understand the dynamics that may have led up to the event, I had no success. Some hypotheses fit but most didn't, as I tried to find new footing in my topsy-turvy life as a grieving single mom.

After several months, I reached an understanding about the event – about people, really. The husband that I thought had an emotional and behavioral range from A to C, from love to anger, actually had a much larger range that I didn't recognize: from A to P, from love to physical abuse. How could I have known? My conclusion: It is impossible to know what someone was truly feeling deep inside or was ultimately capable; *therefore*, I can no longer trust my own perceptions or the behaviors of others. I felt severed from my own grounding.

Mine is a dramatic story of surprise and abuse, but at times our lives *are* dramatic and surprising; many people have experienced much worse. But it is a clear illustration of how native feeling and thought get misinterpreted by a life-changing experience and the pursuit of a new and fitting logic. Similar to Little Albert's story, where an initially soft fuzzy rabbit comes to elicit a fearful response, our manufactured emotions, thoughts, and conclusions get layered atop native experience: we call it emotional baggage.

But as life changes, our conditioned emotions and thoughts often lose their usefulness. In my case, I found it hard to trust close relationships. The native excitement of a new relationship became foreshadowed by the manufactured emotions and thoughts from a decade earlier. It took a lot of counseling to sort out the events and separate my conditioned emotions from my here-and-now native experience, but I did.

Over time, it took learning for my mind to unlearn my programmed emotions and even more time to gain a bit of mastery over sorting out and managing outdated thoughts. It took the willingness to root through paired emotions and thoughts, uncover my flawed logic, and create more realistic knowledge of human behavior, person by person. I had to relearn how to allow myself to re-open to the experience of native feelings and thoughts, but once I did fresh areas of experience opened up around me. I welcomed an improved clarity of thought.

As adults, we often attend to our conditioned responses as though they were real, even a long time after an event has occurred. To avoid painful mental replays, we often cover ourselves in a protective gauze of mindless thought chatter and miss out on our real experience. Our incessant mental chatter serves as a loving nudge from our minds that a deeper truth needs to be known.

Each time we learn a lesson, we replace a fiction with a truth. We come to understand that emotion is only a data point, an invitation to explore an illusion and return to our native experience. Each emotional quest we conquer strengthens our clarity of mind.

Our job, should we take it, is to chase down our manufactured emotions, burst our mythologies of the past, and live into the clarity of mind. Consider it a game of virtual reality, where we look at our lives through the goggles of our past. The emotions are real, the experiences are vivid, and the challenges steep. Some may mistake the game for reality and never turn off their powerful effects. However, we absolutely have the ability to remove our goggles and learn the lessons the stories were meant to teach.

What, then, is wellness of the mind? What are we looking for on the Path of Wellness when it comes to our emotions and thoughts? We are looking for the courage to challenge our emotional assumptions, to recognize that many of our thoughts as are illogical and outdated, and to seek the truth that is always available to us in native experience, in our here-and-now lives.

The experience of The Bog is not an easy one. It is easy to get stuck, go in circles from emotion into faulty logic and back again, and get stuck in the muck. But as we slowly sort our way through the Bog again and again, we build up our muck-raking skills and emerge with a clear and informed mind. What once seemed like overwhelming heartache and challenge has become pressed into the precious gems of lessons learned; these nuggets of hard-earned life are now valuable learnings to share with fellow travelers.

Endearment of Spirit

As we turn our attention to the most mystical aspect of ourselves, our spirit, we are gazing at the Grandest Mystery of all mankind. As we gaze upward toward the heavens, or inward to our deepest sense of self, it creates a sense of awe that we rarely tire of. Spirit exists universally as well as at a deeply personal level. It is natural and flawless, and the wise Alchemist is attuned to its language.

To many, the concept of Spirit can be quite difficult to understand. Religious scholars or philosophers might say that it is not something that can be understood; rather, it is an experience or a state of expanded and heightened consciousness. Early Kabbalists, our ancient mystics, considered it a merging of universal energy, or vibration, with our deepest knowing selves.

We will look first at our universal experience of spirit, something perhaps you call nature, the universe, or God, or "all that is" – the exact word you use is far less important than the understanding of the idea: the realization that energy is the fundamental component of the universe and we all experience it. All matter is composed of electrical vibrations: the earth, the sun, the moon and stars – even ourselves. Every object and every person emits vibration – there are no exceptions. Both animate and inanimate alike emit vibration; our brainwaves, our cells, our thoughts, our physical movements all emit vibration. The atoms that make up a chair are in perpetual vibration.

In a similar vein, everything receives vital energy from neighboring objects. Mountains erode as they give their soil to the river's current and the blowing wind; clouds float in response to currents in the air. Our ears pick up vibration, as do our feet; the blood circulating throughout our bodies responds to pressure in our arteries, it can be felt. Everything in our universe, large and small, is teeming with energy.

This never-ending experience of vibration can be considered "Source" energy, the universal vibration of all that is outside of us. It is more expansive than we can imagine, yet we experience it in the physical environment We are always plugged in to the Universe; we are always receiving and emitting information, whether or not we are aware of it. There is so much Universal vibrational energy, we can't even begin to grasp its enormity.

Vibration is powerful stuff. Perhaps you remember the 7.2 Richter magnitude Great East Japan Earthquake in 2011 that had such a large vibrational impact that it triggered tsunami waves over 133 feet high; the vibration moved the island of Japan eight feet to the east, shifted the earth on its axis by ten feet, and generated sound waves so large they were picked up by low-orbiting satellites.

In contrast, consider the wings of a butterfly fluttering in the breeze. There, too, vibrations are emitted, which are received by the sensitive receptors of plants and animals, registering slight variation in the environment as they attend to the movement. If a butterfly were to flutter near our cheek, we might experience a very slight vibration and sit back in awe that we just felt the breeze of butterfly wings.

As we encounter our worlds, our bodies pick up vibration from sources near and far from us that are there to be "heard," or received, depending upon the sensitivity of our body. We register Source energy as vibration, but our minds and spirit are the blank slates left to interpret the vibration into something meaningful to our minds.

"Source" energy is the singular vibration of the Universe in each of us; it creates worlds, ignites the imagination, sparks thought, and births inspiration. It is generated outside our bodies and penetrates within our physical boundaries. Our skin, our boundary to the world, is semi-permeable, and we are superb receptors. As expert vibrational translators, we learn to interpret millions of vibrations in our environment and begin to decipher their meaning in our lives.

"Spirit" is our *individual* experience of source energy. It is the life energy, what the Taoists call "Chi," within us that fuels our bodies and our minds. As Source energy teems outside of us, we translate the information we are receiving. Who is the translator, the "I" that gives it meaning? As we think about awareness, we have the concept of the "experiencer" versus that part of our selves that responds to the awareness and knowledge of the experience – the clear, objective observer. We hold a boundary inside our own non-physical experience between what is being experienced and our deeper observing selves.

Many years ago, I was in a car accident where I nearly went through the passenger-side windshield. I can recall a very clear awareness after the impact with another car as a thought that said, "You are going to go through the windshield." The statement was very clear, concise, and focused; strictly factual. As microseconds can, at times of trauma, be experienced as long seconds, this moment contained a very clear awareness, a very simple observation, that given the movement of my body at the point of impact, my trajectory inside the car was through the glass. That was it. *Awareness* of the moment, complete. The observer had translated the vibrations of sound, movement, of my legs sliding across the front seat. Done; data received.

Then a second voice piped in, "Oh no, I don't want to go through the windshield!" It was a *feeling* of dread; I didn't want that experience. There was a very clear demarcation between the observation of the collision and the feeling associated with the processing of the event. The observer and the experiencer. Spirit's observation of events and my reaction to it.

Fortunately, my body stopped short of contact with the glass, but my recollection of the experience has been vivid in my mind ever since. It was a formative experience where I could clearly distinguish the boundary between my observer and the experiencer of the event.

Who was the observer? The observer was "Spirit," total awareness before native feeling and thought intervened. Pure innate reception and knowledge, separate and apart from any reaction to it such as "This can't be good." This is a very important distinction to be made within ourselves; it is our direct experience of Spirit that is operating within us at all times. At times we are fortunate enough to experience Spirit in slow, precise motion – it is a remarkable and memorable event. Most of the time, unfortunately, we take it for granted or are unaware of it altogether.

We all have access to our observer at any time we wish to feel direct contact with Spirit. Simply pause and quiet your thinking mind. Find a comfortable spot – in nature is ideal – and slowly look around you. Rest in the comfort of your native experience, notice your native feelings or thoughts apart from your knowing self. It may take a little practice, but you will eventually learn to make the distinction between your observer, your Spirit, and everything else. Relish in the awe of this marvelous capacity that rests with our own skins.

This is Spirit, this is you, the driver on life's journey, the fountainhead of your inspiration.

Not only does Spirit observe, it also provides loving guidance. Have you ever asked yourself "What do I do next?" and a gentle mental voice within answers with support and guidance? Perhaps you recognize this voice as your conscience, your inner wisdom. Notice that this voice is *always* loving and supportive. Ask your inner self, your Spirit, a question and listen for the answer. It will come because you have asked.

Our sense of Spirit also shows up in our daily lives. Have you ever had a stunning idea that pops into your mind and you know it as intuitively correct, a gut instinct? It is the spark of intuition – Spirit merging with Source energy the moment they come in contact. Some might call it divine inspiration.

This is a technique I use when writing poetry. I might gaze into nature, usually the yard outside my living room window, quiet my native experience and thinking mind (yes, it can be done), and allow nature and spirit to mix together directly. I write down the resulting words, whatever they are, and voilà! Poetry.

Spirit is also our origination point of inspiration, the point of inception letting us know through desire our next idea, our next step. It has the quality of "of course-ness." One day, in a brainstorming session, several of us were exploring how to capture the "Ah-ha's" of our seminar participants. One team member popped up and down like a popcorn kernel and exclaimed, "We could have a tree of "Ah-ha's!" It was intuitively right, the perfect inspiration, a divine gift of the merging of Source energy (coming from the group's search for answers) and Spirit. The moment the idea became voice the whole team sat in silent astonishment – Spirit was dancing with Source.

This is *you*, Spirit creating, Source energy and Spirit merging to give voice to a new reality. This *is* how we create the world, how cities get built, how lives are saved through medical invention. This is Source energy at its best, merging with individual Spirit, giving birth to idea and idea becoming reality.

Rest in your own pure knowing, marvel with your divine inspiration as Source meets Spirit. Create that world that yearns to be built. We all have this remarkable process going on all day, every day. Find it in yourself and honor it as the divinity that it is.

Mastery of Environment

Living into inspiration requires us to consider the environment we live in. As you stroll through your environment, you will notice its inherent beauty, from trees whose green leaves open your heart to the brilliance of nature, to the sounds of the birds or insects that bring sweetness to your ears. You experience the fresh, fragrant smell of a recent rain that seems to lift your emotions to the renewal of the environment around you. How refreshing! On that very same stroll, however, you might find areas littered with beer cans and candy wrappers. Perhaps the people nearby are making noises that disturb your solitude and ruin the experience of the beauty around you.

Every day we "dance" with our environment; perhaps we brace against the wind, slow down in the heat, or withdraw in a tense environment. This dance is a crucial source of – or impediment to – our wellness. The personal impact of our environment is globally under-esteemed as a significant factor of wellness.

The overall health of our environment is part of the dance, and impacts our wellness in several ways. We are aware more than ever that global warming threatens our existence; we know that auto and industrial exhaust poison our air and pesticides and antibiotics invade our well-balanced bodies. We do our best to cope, including driving through legislation to preserve our environment or adjusting our diets to be more healthful. As with most things, we as individuals cope differently, and react to changes in our environment as best as we can.

When I was young, I often experienced nearly debilitating anxiety when I commuted to work along a busy freeway. I often had to pull off the road to gather myself. Although I didn't mind the congested freeways, this particular journey through the Quagmire seemed unusually treacherous.

I never really understood why my anxiety was so pronounced until decades later, when I traveled through the old neighborhood. The echo of decades-old anxiety once again pumped through my every cell, broadcasting its warnings. It was then that I inhaled the vision of the town where I had worked, a gang-ridden, industrial part of Los Angeles where the pollution was thick and the crime was high. Through my years of experience, I had come to understand the permeability of self, that environments unfriendly to my natural calm could infuse my experience and overwhelm my sensitivities. It was in that moment I understood the ineffable influence of body, mind, and spirit *with* the environment.

As travelers journeying through the Quagmire, nature has equipped us with the ability to dance with our environment, to move and experience ourselves in synchronicity with that which surrounds us. How do we dance with our environment? Biology has taught us that the air that we breathe, chemicals, solid objects (the "stuff" around us), and our bodies, organs, and cells are all made up of atoms and different combinations of molecules, and that the space between molecules and atoms is vast, at least in relative terms. Physics further tells us that solidity is relative, too, with some objects being denser or more permeable than others.

Our eyes, ears, nose, mouth, and skin are sensitive receptors. Being vibrationally adept receivers, both obvious and more subtle aspects of our environment are always known to us at some level. We are not usually aware of such nuance, yet our environment bombards us with information day and night. We feel tense when others around us are in conflict; we cringe at the sight of moldy food in our refrigerator which reminds us of degrees of neglect. We feel delight in the presence of innocent youth, or in the experience of emotional spaciousness as we drive from urban sprawl to country roads. What is outside our physical boundaries permeates our inner experience.

Managing the dance is key to wellness. As I drove through industrial, crime-infused Los Angeles the environment's vibration, its chemicals and its fearful vibes, penetrated my experience. Once I became aware of my own permeability to the environment, of the infusion of unwelcome sights, sounds, and vibes into my otherwise peaceful experience, a new dimension of reality became apparent to me. I could feel it, I could name it, and I could now manage my experience of it.

We are all affected by our environments. Our surroundings quietly influence our physical, emotional, and spiritual experience. Have you ever noticed the shift in your experience after you have cleaned up a messy desk or a cluttered kitchen? Our environment makes a big difference on our well-being.

As we trek through the Quagmire, we quickly find that each path offers its own unique reality. Perhaps the weather is hot and humid.

Perhaps you are sensitive to the heat and humidity and are hindered by the climate, yet others around you find a way to adapt. Perhaps we shed a layer of clothing or follow along in the shaded, tree-lined areas. After a while we become familiarized, or acclimated, to the environment.

In a similar way, we encounter and adapt to the people we meet on the Path of Wellness – our social environment. People around us have a tremendous influence on our well-being. Perhaps they are short encounters, or perhaps they are the people we live with or work with. I am very sensitive to my husband's vibes. When he is highly stressed, the energy he throws off is very intense and difficult for me to be around. I often need to go read a book in a different room. Yet his friends easily vibrate at this level and experience little if any difficulty. On the other hand, at times my husband's energy is smooth, grounded, and calm, and he forms the perfect shape sitting next to me on the couch. He is then a perfect complement to our lovely space.

Imagine how the people in your environment affect your emotional or spiritual life. Are some people easy to be around, while others present overwhelming challenges? These are experiences to become aware of and learn how to manage.

It is not my intention in this book to provide relationship coaching; however, I do want to convey how important other people are to our own environmental well-being and how they can add to, or detract from, our health and wellness.

Learning how to dance with our environment is a key element to our well-being. We can clean it up, change it out, or adorn it to complement our innermost beauty. But make no mistake: it will make a difference in your wellness.

I encourage you to look around your house, your office, your car, your city, or your world and imagine a perfect place or a perfect space. We have the *choice* to build our environment any way we wish. We can create it to recover our innate qualities of love and tenderness: for example, we can add natural beauty with gardens and houseplants, enact laws to preserve our environment and our food supply, and we can choose to exit those environments that are not healthy for us.

We also have the choice *not* to act; a choice rarely, if ever, valued on the Path of Wellness.

~

It has been several decades since I began the Quest for Wellness, having had remarkable results. After my first three years of illness, I met a seaworthy Alchemist. He ran lots of tests, talked to me at length, and pronounced me has having a "lifestyle disease." There were several long medical words describing how my lifestyle affected my wellness, but none of them mattered. At that point, my body had given way to its altered chemistry, and it took a unique mix of experimental treatment, balanced life practices, and an insistent spiritual desire to be normal and alter the course of my life.

I hope this chapter has helped you more clearly distinguish the essential four aspects of ourselves – body, mind, spirit, and environment – and encouraged you to explore each one independently of the others. This is only intended to be a practice, a strengthening of the ability to see each in its own light without interference from the others. Play with them, experiment, and learn their different qualities and how they arise uniquely in you. You will need those skills in Part II, as you learn to masterfully combine them and live into your inspiration.

You need only one other thing before you continue on the Path of Wellness: you must know who you are.

~

Reflecting on your thoughts about body, mind, spirit and environment – all that you have done to get your needs met in the Quagmire – you know that you have lived a long life in pursuit of your Grand

Mystery, posed many Big Questions, and have undertaken many Quests. You have stepped forward, and sometimes backward, countless times; you have explored uncharted territory, won many battles, and learned from mistakes.

"I have always been on a journey," you reminisce, "I will begin just where I should – with today!"

Then, from some deeply intimate place, rustling from within, you hear the voice of your own wisdom:

"There is nothing to change, no places to go back to, and nothing to fix. All that lies before you is awareness, consciousness, inspiration, and the next step. It's all good."

Alchemist's Practice

The Alchemist of Experience develops an *astute understanding* of their own body, mind, spirit, and environment; able to identify each *aspect* of themselves as individual components of "self". They begin to look at the characteristics, or qualities, of each and become knowledgeable about how they experience them in their lives. The Alchemist, without judgment, also becomes an expert at tuning into "here-and-now" *native experience* and is able to extract out conditioned thoughts and feelings. They know that mastery of their experience takes practice, and they are willing to take the time and make the effort to prepare themselves for the journey through the Quagmire. The Alchemist's Grand Mystery is always calling them forward.

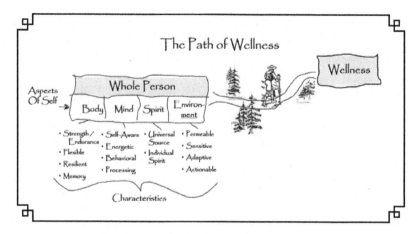

1. **Focus on Body** – Find a quiet, comfortable location to sit. You can sit on a chair or on the floor, whatever is most comfortable for you. Close your eyes and begin to take long, slow inhales and exhales. Bring your attention to your breath, notice how your chest rises and falls with each. Sit quietly for about a minute, then imagine bringing your breath into your legs. Perhaps you can feel some tingling, a heaviness, or other sensation in your legs or toes. After five breath cycles, move your attention and your breath upward to your arms. Notice how your arms are placed and what sensations you experience in your forearms, your wrists, or your fingers. After five breath cycles, move your attention and your breath to your head. Do you experience sensations in your head? Perhaps your head is weighty, your facial muscles are relaxed, or your jaw is tensed. Take the time to slowly notice and become aware of all part of of your body.

2. **Focus on Enviroment** – Sit quietly for a few more moments, then gently open your eyes. Gaze about the room slowly. Gently draw your gaze to any object nearby and become aware as to whether the object brings forth a pleasing feeling or something less pleasing. Can you notice the quick spark of a thought? Gently, let the experience go.

Repeat this activity on another object (or objects) in the room. Become aware of the feeling the object brings forth, and perhaps the quick thought that goes along with it.

3. **Focus on Mind** – Continuing to sit quietly, think of the next person you are likely to see. Maybe it is a family member, or a friend or coworker. Sit quietly for about two minutes thinking about this person. Notice your thoughts about this person. Are they positive or negative? Do you imagine a conversation, or perhaps remember a previous incident? Let your thoughts and feelings flow freely; there is no need to censor yourself.

4. **Focus on Spirit** – Come back to sitting quietly in your chair or otherwise comfortable location, gently close your eyes again, and return your attention to your breath. Continue to breathe in long slow inhales and exhales, and when you are ready, see if you can mentally picture yourself sitting in the chair. Just *notice* the experience, don't stop to think. Then return your attention to your breath. Practice this exercise a few times, each time through seeing whether you can observe yourself in the room.

5. Once again, return your attention to your breathing and bring your attention back into the room around you. Sit quietly for a few minutes; then prepare to make a few notes on your experience.

6. Describe how you experienced each Aspect of yourself during each part of the exercise. Note how you can describe one aspect of yourself apart from the others. Could you distinguish significant differences between body, mind, spirit, and environment? During the Practice, what did you experience? Or Feel? Or Think? Notice if you didn't experience much of anything – that is an important experience, as well.

Make some notes below; record your experiences, practice putting words to them. Become familiar with each unique aspect of yourself. Pay close attention to the subtle differences. (You may need a journal!)

NOTES:

My Body

_____

_____

_____

_____

My Mind

_____

_____

_____

_____

My sense of spirit

_____

_____

_____

My environment

_____

_____

_____

_____

Write it down, put words to it. Find the subtle. (Find a journal!)

∞

Chapter 3

~

The Role of the Alchemist

*"We create wellness – our vibrational energy of
desire and inspiration is an ever-present given."*
–J. K. S. Zetlan

~

*Mind no longer appears to be an accidental
intruder into the realm of matter...we ought
rather hail it as the creator and governor of the
realm of matter."*

–Sir James Jean, 1930

You have been traveling for a very long time: it's hard to tell if it has
been hours or even days. At times you feel sluggish, but often you
feel as though you have traveled to a much stronger place than
when you began (whenever that was!). The Path of Wellness is quite
beautiful. There are plenty of shaded trees to sit under if you need to
stop for a rest, but the trek is steep.

As you begin to ascend a rocky embankment, you notice that the
Path of Wellness is thick with travelers. You can hear the heavy
breathing of a few out-of-breath travelers as they pass you by; but
several ahead of you appear to be turning back. Perhaps you are
going in the wrong direction!

"Excuse me," you say to a fellow sojourner that has paused for a rest along the incline, "I am on the Path of Wellness; how do I know if I am going in the right direction?"

"I see," said the hiker as she twirls a pirouette and points up the path, "since you can only go ahead or backward on this route, it is truly up to you to decide. Perhaps you should consult the Alchemist."

"The who?" you ask.

~

Meet the Alchemist

As we embark upon the Path of Wellness, we often wonder "How do I know that I'm moving forward? How can I be certain that I am directionally correct?" This is when you must meet the Alchemist. The Alchemist is a wise soul and carries very special tools.

- ✓ *Measurement* – to discern how far one has traveled;

- ✓ *Compass* – to ensure one is headed in the right direction;

- ✓ *A Radar Instrument (Debris Wiper)* – to detect and avoid potential dangers.

As you travel great distances and grow on your journey, you observe many things. The sunrise. The sunset. The mountains with their lush greenery, large and small, tall and round. You also learn many things about the sun, the moon, and how the tides and the seasons affect you. You meet fellow travelers and learn much about them. You observe how communities come together, and how beliefs and attitudes can shape the world. You experience the miracles of technology, enabling you to feel someone's emotions from continents away, and to easily travel to places on the other side of the globe.

You learn so much, yet you find that you also know so little. Perhaps in your more mystical moments you wonder how this incredible universal machine came into being and how it somehow all works together; the tides and the moon, the seasons and their harvests; your life, and the lives of those you love. How has this all come to pass and, specifically, who are you in the matter of it all?

In the golden hours of dawn, you come upon a small lake in a lush meadow. Stooping beside the glass-smooth surface of the water to ponder its depths, you take in the grandeur of the surrounding mountains, the iron-brown richness of the soil, and the gentle ripples of the water as it laps against shore. Your gaze is quietly drawn into the eyes of the lake as you exchange an unfamiliar yet knowing look. Staring transfixed at the water's reflection you see, for the first time, the eyes of who can only be the master of your universe, the Alchemist.

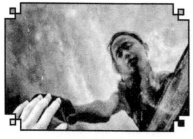

It is here, gazing into the eyes of the lake, that you realize that you are the creator of your own life, *you* are the Alchemist. *You* set out on this journey to learn about your Grand Mystery. *You* are asking the Big Questions, and *you* chose this path to the lake. *You* have discovered that you alone have the tools to sense your environment and chart your course. You are the receptor and the emitter, the source of information, the antennae of your radar, the driver and the navigator. To be successful in your journey, you must learn how to combine the key elements of perception and knowledge to chart your destiny. The role of someone who combines these diverse elements to create something of value is *you*, the Alchemist.

The Role of the Alchemist

Have you ever wondered how you got here? Who is pulling the oars that propel us, and who measures the winds to set the direction that got you where you are today? Many of us were raised to believe we are a byproduct of our environment, growing to become responsible adults, yet the challenge of gaining self-understanding to fully embrace all that you hope to become has been left entirely to you.

Our wellness, our inspiration, the currents of thoughts, feelings, and emotions that flow within us sometimes appear to change by whimsy, and often those around us bring forward Big Questions. It is up to each one of us to learn as much as possible about how we, in general, and *you*, specifically, perceive, process, and navigate the life that you have *right now*. You must learn to be the "Alchemist" of your own experience to more fully understand your life today and to enable you to create your future through inspiration.

It may seem mysterious, but learning the role of the Alchemist is actually quite simple. Simply put, Alchemy *is taking what you learn about yourself and applying it in a way that causes you to experience relief, or pleasure.*

For example, the feeling of anger in some people actually covers up a deeper feeling of fear. What if you took that valuable piece of information and asked yourself one of the Big Questions: "What am I afraid of?" Years ago, when my husband and I began to date, I would notice that women were drawn to him, enjoying his attention. I found myself often jealous or angry, those feelings often surfacing either directly, or to my own embarrassment, indirectly. Living on a daily diet of fear and jealousy was a very negative experience, so I asked myself that Big Question: "What am I afraid of?" The quick response: "Losing this relationship." I felt "less than" many of the other women, so I began a quest to become a loving, supportive, intelligent, and caring partner. I deeply desired to make him happy (deeply true for me), and I also knew my behavior was counter to who I wished to become. Bit by bit, I began to change my behavior to come into alignment with my authentic desire, learning to choose love over reaction and to offer trust instead of suspicion. Whenever I noticed a negative reaction, I found a way to come back into my "here-and-now" experience and express myself in a loving and supportive way. It wasn't easy, and I worked hard to get it done.

We must all make adjustments in life to live into the best version of ourselves. We learn something about ourselves and make a change for the better. We all do this; however, there are two skills the Alchemist of Experience uses that most people don't exercise: 1) they build an ever-deepening understanding of human experience; and 2) they make clear adjustments in themselves that are in *alignment* with the *futures* that inspire them.

Understanding the human experience takes a willingness to study and learn about how people work and then testing what you learn to see if it is true for *you*. If it's true for you, use it and keep learning. If it's not a fit, don't use it and continue learning. There are bookstores, ebooks, YouTube videos, and blogs about the experience of being human. In addition, you can read from the ancients, Buddhism, the Tao Te Ching, or something from your own spiritual underpinnings. You can read the sciences; pick up a psychology book, explore the nature of consciousness from various sources. The more you learn and test, the greater your ability to understand yourself and effect positive change in your life. You are putting tools of knowledge into your *Alchemist's Toolkit*.

Finally, Alchemists test what they have learned and then find the shortest direct route to their dreams. To do this, Alchemists are sensitive to the currents in their lives – body, mind, spirit, and environment – and are guided by their Great Mystery, their deepest yearnings of what they would like to affect during their time on this earth.

As you journey through this book, you have already begun to master your experience. You have started to build a firm and steady grounding based on Core Beliefs and have come to the Path of Wellness. You now have learned that the Alchemist develops a tried-and-tested toolkit of knowledge and actively applies that knowledge to realize his/her deepest yearnings. Yet there is one additional bit of science that sits at the very root of the Alchemist's knowledge.

The Alchemist's Science

Although alchemy was debunked centuries ago as false science, the Alchemist of today looks to science for scientific validation for what we intuitively know. Recent discoveries in physics are uncovering the science of what the ancients have understood for thousands of years: that we humans are composed of vibrational energy. The ancient Zohar described the universe as "...permeated by spiritual forces endlessly circulating...." Modern science, through quantum mechanics, has been able to observe our "spiritual forces" and has defined them in terms of electromagnetism, the force derived from the presence, motion, and attraction of charged particles – our energies.

In 1930, Sir James Jeans, Professor of Applied Mathematics, Physics, and Astronomy at Cambridge and Princeton Universities, made stunning contributions to the field of quantum mechanics by flipping our understanding of "self" and the world on its head. In his book, *The Mysterious Universe*, Jeans writes:

> *"The stream of knowledge is heading towards a non-mechanical reality; the Universe begins to look more like a great thought than like a great machine. Mind no longer appears to be an accidental intruder into the realm of matter...we ought rather hail it as the creator and governor of the realm of matter."*

As recently as 2005, Richard Cohn Henry, professor at the Henry A. Rowland Department of Physics and Astronomy at John Hopkins University, wrote a landmark essay in the prestigious journal *Nature* entitled "The Mental Universe". He scientifically supports Jeans' research, noting that "bright physicists [today are] again led to believe the unbelievable – this time that the world is mental."

The more we study, the more we continue to evolve our thinking about who we really are. We are beginning to comprehend that we are Creators, rather than the Created. This is a profound change in the understanding of "self" that enables us to change our thinking about our own lives. We need to be like Galileo, who, in the fifteenth century, reversed popular opinion about how we understood the universe. He proved through geometric physics and astronomy that the Earth goes around the Sun. In a similar manner, science is now beginning to better understand our own role in creating our lives, and the results are not what most of us were taught.

The Alchemist learns from the wisdom of the ancients, but also accepts scientific insight. The fact that we are vibrational energy, in the scientific sense, enables us to manage our world of matter and belief through thought, including our desires and inspiration. It turns out that we are vibrational spirits with kinetic bodies, and co-creators of our world. Thoughts that begin as this vibrational energy filter down into our hearts and minds and become inspiration. It is our inspiration that creates worlds, from metaphysical feelings to the physical, including roads, skyscrapers, cities, and more.

As Alchemists, we create the very substance of our lives. Through our thoughts and the actions that result from them, Alchemists can create the positive aspects of our lives, including jobs, families, communities, and even our own personae. We can create wellness and inspiration. But Alchemists can also create negative aspects of our lives, resulting in suffering, pain or sickness, and our fanciful illusions.

Although ancient mystics understood this thousands of years ago, they kept most of it silent – it was knowledge before its time, an understanding that was out of sync with the thinking of their age. As we journey through the Quagmire we will continue to "pull a Galileo" on the proven nature of self by knowing, and even testing, that we are the Creators, not simply the created.

The Alchemist's Toolkit

With our Grand Mystery awaiting us on the horizon, and our choice to achieve wellness affirmed, we will certainly want to know where we stand today in relation to our intended goals. How do you know that you are moving forward on your quests and are traveling in the right direction? If you lose a step or two, what tools do you have to ensure that you can resume your journey in the right direction?

As was mentioned in the earlier part of this chapter, there are three tools in the Alchemist's toolkit: it is important to know more about them. They include:

+ The *Alchemist's Measure* – is a length or line that is typically marked at regular intervals. It is used to draw straight lines and measure direction and distance on a journey or quest.

+ The *Language of Well-Being* – is a descriptive vocabulary that informs the Alchemist where they are when beginning a journey and is used to ensure they are moving forward on the crest of inspiration – a type of compass based in language.

+ The *Radar Instrument* – is a sensitive mechanism, our whole self, that is used to gather navigational information about the ease or difficulty of a quest, and which helps direct us to the easiest route possible.

The Alchemist's Measure

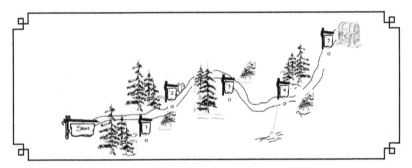

Imagine we are on a long trail that we know is a five-mile, one-way outing, as pictured here. At the end of the trail is a treasure where you will find the answer to one of your Big Questions. Along the path are mile markers that let you know how far you have traveled, and which enable you to understand the distance to the destination. The trail may be seen as your Measure, the mile markers as milestones that gauge the distance traveled. Each time you pass a mile marker that shows a higher number, you confirm that you are going in the right direction.

Dieting uses such a measurement system. If your target weight is 130, and you now weigh 150, you have twenty pounds to lose to reach your target weight. If you lose fifteen pounds you know you are going in the *right direction*. If you then gain five pounds you know you are backsliding a little bit, going *somewhere else* other than your target. At that point you can reaffirm your intention and resume losing weight.

If however, you start your diet weighing 150 pounds, with a target of 130, and you weigh in at 155, you know you are going *somewhere else*, in the wrong direction, and you can then reevaluate your intention for weight loss and choose to get on a better weight loss path.

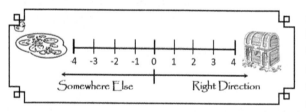

As the sum total of our wellness, we might think of ourselves somewhere along a continuum, or your Alchemist's Measure. At the far left of the continuum we might find illness, or another undesirable condition; at the far right absolute vitality. Perhaps in the middle we feel OK (and holding a steady path), and while we may occasionally feel better or worse, we are generally doing OK.

As we measure wellness, we sometimes have objective measures to help us chart our way, like blood pressure, calcium, blood sugar, etc., where we can clearly mark our improvements based on a healthy range of test results. However, sometimes the measures are entirely subjective. Alchemists also measure feelings, emotions, attitudes, and thoughts. Using the *Alchemist's Measure*, you can understand where you are on the continuum between hope and anger, or between the sense of fear and joy. Wellness is *always* in the direction of things that please, that feel good. Feelings, thoughts, and attitudes are as subjectively measurable as physical measures and can help guide us on our journey.

Finally, our environment has both objective and subjective elements that can be placed along a measured wellness continuum. Things like smog, drought, and temperature are discretely measurable using scientifically proven methods. But the mountains, your back yard, your office, or the appeal of the city you live in each has a personal, subjective measure of beauty, expansion, pleasure, and wellness.

As we travel in the overall direction of wellness, and ultimately into living an inspired life, the Alchemist uses the *Measure* as a treasured indicator of *choice and direction*. For example, using the Alchemists *Measure*, have you chosen wellness, or something else? Have you back-slid in an area (my office is a mess!), or have you taken strides in the direction of wellness (do I feel more in control of my space)? All directions of movement, forward and backward, are choices; they are not accidental and they are not imposed by outside forces. The *Alchemist's Measure* is that measure of choice; the choice to live into your Core Beliefs, the choice to live into Wellness and the choice to live into an inspired life.

The Language of Well-Being

How would you describe your journey through the Quagmire? Is it treacherous, hard and full of potholes? Or is it a piece of cake with all the servings and frosting you'd like? The words we use in our speech, both out loud to others and internally to ourselves, convey our thoughts, feelings, and experience to deliver messages. As in writing a story, we choose words for the impact they produce on the reader, including the emotions and feelings that we wish to convey. Our words and our thoughts are electromagnetic packets of energy that deliver an energetic message. They have intensity, frequency, and duration. They are also directional; they can be positive, negative, or neutral. Our words create visual imagery within our mind's eye which are similar to a picture we either want to hang on our wall or hide in a closet.

Here are a few examples of how words can affect us. What feeling tone or imagery do they bring to mind?

> *"The year that Bibi turned ten, which was twelve years before Death came calling on her, the sky was a grim vault of sorrow...and the angles cried down flood upon flood...the days and nights washed by the grief of angles."*
>
> *—Dean Koontz, Ashley Bell*
>
> *"It was the language of enthusiasm, of things accomplished with love and purpose..."*
>
> *—Paulo Coelho, The Alchemist*
>
> *"The opinion of this so-called judge...is ridiculous and will be overturned!"*
>
> *—Donald J. Trump*

Words are important. They direct our thoughts and frame our values and attitudes, they create and perpetuate stories – whether true or not. They can negatively charge a relationship, or authenticate a deep and caring feeling. Each and every word we speak delivers a positive or negative vibrational message both the speaker and the listener take to heart.

As receptive listeners, we tend to believe what we hear. We listen to our parents praise or criticize us, and we believe their statements to be true. We learn that "It's a hard life," or that "Life is a smorgasbord." The words played across the airways soon become reality whether they are true or not. The words we speak to ourselves become reality as well, whether true or not. Everyone in proximity to the words we hear receives their vibrational message and we are compelled to do *something* with them.

The words we speak deliver intention. Some words are intended to influence, some are meant to share ideas or to defend a point of view. Words can uplift and create a positive energetic environment, and other words deliver anger or hate. We say the things we do for very precise reasons, and, through our language, we give shape to our lives and often to the lives of others. Unfortunately, most of us don't weigh our intentions and choose our words wisely in day-to-day conversation; we tend to be sloppy speakers and partial listeners. Yet when it comes to living an inspired life, the words you use and hear matter as you walk the path towards the Inspired Life.

I remember that when I was a budding yoga instructor, I felt embarrassed as I stumbled over providing clear direction, using poetic speech and speaking Sanskrit. I would hear myself say something incorrectly, and my eyes and mouth would pinch together in personal annoyance. What was I telling myself at that moment? My thoughts were "You are a terrible teacher," "You should know this stuff by now," and other unkind and untrue messages.

I began to work on my own negative self-talk. Honestly, I truly *was* a new instructor. Every word out of my mouth was a learning opportunity, and I seized every opportunity to listen to my words and make better selections. I began to think as an artist selecting words that provided my desired feeling tone in the room, words that supported and uplifted struggling students and also uplifted me. This is how I began to change my self-talk.

Those initial automatic words I was speaking to myself had power; they were intensely negative, and I would think those negative thoughts for long periods of time. They made me feel bad, depleted my energy, and made me mimic other instructors rather than find my own voice. They did real harm. But as I changed my internal language, my opinion of myself underwent radical change. I started with a more positive point of view of "instructor-ness as a journey," and used incrementally more uplifting language. Today the words I use in a class bring the student much farther along than simple narrative instruction. My self-talk is uplifting and inspires me to consider how I want to grow next. My own words healed. The *Language of Inspiration* is an important resource in the Alchemist's Toolkit.

As packets of energies, words have positive and negative charges; they have polar opposites like hate/love, fear/confidence, joy/sadness, delight/displeasure. Some words have stronger charges than others, such as satisfy vs. relish, or stir vs. electrify, or irritate vs. enrage. Using the *Language of Wellness*, and knowing that we tend to believe our words, the Alchemist uses language as a tool.

Used as a tool, language is a compass – an *indicator of direction*. Imagine that as you begin your journey down the Path of Wellness you come upon a second traveler sitting beside the trail. After you share a warm "Hello," the traveler looks you squarely in the eye and begins to tell you how hard the path is, that it has been poorly kept (it has caused him to fall more than once), that the journey wasn't worth the effort after all, and, besides, it's rainy out and he does not wish to ruin his new shoes.

What does the Alchemist conclude?

The Alchemist listens to the words the traveler has spoken and notices, at first glance, that there are six negative references in the hiker's description: "hard," "poorly kept," "caused him," "wasn't worth the effort," "besides," "ruin." Among the negative words, there were zero positive references, not even a "hello." The Alchemist concludes that this is an unhappy person and, given his negative state of mind, is surely going to return to his starting point in the Quagmire. For this traveler, the journey has been a trudge, surely not a positive direction. After all, the Alchemist reasons, this is just a path with nature doing what nature does. And the rain – it's doing its job; it keeps the shrubs nourished and may quench his thirst further down the path.

Feeling a bit of compassion for the discouraged traveler and noting the traveler hasn't yet learned the *Language of Inspiration*, the Alchemist resumes his journey. By now the rain is smelling sweet, and the muddy soil provides an ideal opportunity to practice footing and balance. Our compass is pointing in a positive direction.

A second thing the Alchemist uses language for is to *create inspiration*. As the Alchemist continues the journey on the Path of Wellness, the urge to eat something trickles up from the stomach and he sits down to enjoy a favorite snack of apples and almonds. He meets a second traveler who is passing by on his way deeper into forest. Stopping to say "Hello," the Alchemist offers this traveler a couple of almonds and a slice of his apple. The traveler begins to share his experience: "It hasn't rained in weeks, and I am so glad the earth is getting nourished. I began to practice my balance a ways back and nearly fell over, but I remembered to keep a strong stance and sit back a bit into my heels. It was awesome! I'm not sure about the trail ahead, but I know with certainty if I keep practicing my balance I will eventually be able to succeed on this muddy trail."

What does the Alchemist conclude from the second traveler's story?

Listening to the traveler's words, we learn that the earth is getting nourished, a simple quest about his own balancing on a muddy trail is in progress and that with a little more practice, he will certainly be able to succeed on the hike. It's interesting to note that the traveler seems enthralled by his experience on the path; it is as if the journey is as much fun as the thought of reaching the destination.

To the Alchemist, the Path of Wellness is an exhilarating challenge, one to be enjoyed, even if there are setbacks. There is much to learn.

The *Language of Inspiration* is full of descriptive words and is easy to understand. Simply by applying the *Alchemist's Measure* to study one's words, it is possible to discern where they are relative to their quest's destination. It is also possible to compare words used yesterday to today's words and tell the direction they are going (hopefully in the "right direction" rather than "someplace else"). In addition, they can select the words they use in the future to increase their wellness and speed up the journey.

Therefore, it is important to note that words can be placed along the *Alchemist's Measure*, from -4 to +4. Minus-4 means you have gone to the extreme end of the undesirable, Zero means you are (just)

OK and Plus-4 indicates that you are fully headed in the desired direction. Using *Language* with the *Measure* to indicate where you are on the Path of Wellness is a good choice. It can also aid in choosing words wisely to create even greater wellness. Try moving up the Language of Wellness scale to reach for a more satisfying, abundant life experience.

The Language of Well-Being

Sample Thoughts, Emotions and Feelings

-4 Rage / Despondent	-3 Angry / Depressed	-2 Annoyed / Disappointed	-1 Doubt / Frustration	0 OKAY	1 Optimism	2 Pleased	3 Happy	4 Love / Appreciation
Grief	Sad	Disappointed	Doubtful	Don't care	Glad	Inspired	Joyful	Ecstatic
Despondent	Depressed	Dissatisfied	Worried	No feelings	Pleased	Satisfied	Confident	Appreciation
Helpless	Angry	Unhappy	Concerned	Okay	Optimistic	Very pleased	Happy	Reverent
Terrified	Frightened	Scared	Frustrated	So-so	Eager	Successful	Strong	Divine
Rage	Rare	Annoyed	Not enough	Fair	Look Forward	Proud	Serene	Love
Hate	Paniced	Missing	Unsettling		Encouraged	Motivated	Calm	Blissful
Impossible		Anxious	Hesitant		Enough	Plenty	Lots	Abundant
					Engaging	Like	Love	In the flow
						Absorbing	Encompasing	

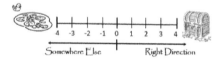

Somewhere Else   Right Direction

Not long ago I had a group of friends visiting my home. We were sitting around the fire on our redwood deck among beautiful shrubbery. People began to share characteristics of themselves they felt were good and valuable. As people began to share about themselves, the conversation revealed a rather disturbing characteristic. One woman began to share about her compassionate side, but her sharing quickly turned into self-criticism; aspects of herself that she didn't like. Others chimed in to analyze why she might be experiencing her hardships, and before long the group began to sympathize and go into analysis about the problem. Analyses like "You know what probably happened…" and "so-and-so was probably thinking…" consumed the conversation. What became apparent was that the group was drawn into a vortex of negativity, analysis paralysis, and rationalization that only served to extend everyone's time and energy in downward spiraling conversation. "Pleased" degraded into "frustrated," which devolved into "unhappy" and then "angry." The entire group went *"someplace else"* rather than in the intended direction of their positive attributes.

Others took turns in sharing their "positive attributes," with each conversation ending up in similar rationalization of why things were bad with many "tsk, tsk's" reaffirming the futility of each situation. During the evening, I sat in suspended disbelief at how the group members supported one another's problems and the Ocean of Despair appeared to grow broader and deeper. Misery does indeed love company.

Listen carefully to yourself and to other travelers along your journey. Observe; take note of the words unwittingly used and the direction in which the conversation is headed. Through observation, learn about the power of language to entrench ourselves on paths going *"somewhere else"* or to extend and broaden our experience on the Path of Wellness. The Language of Wellness is a powerful tool and introduces us to broad vistas of insight and possibility, enticing adventures and ever-increasing joy as we proceed on our journey through the Quagmire – on our quest for Living into Wellness and Inspiration.

The Alchemist's Instrument

Have you ever considered yourself a fine-tuned instrument? We are exactly that. We process the vibration in our environment like a fine-tuned lens. If we know where we are headed, we know whether our current experience is aligned to meet that objective. If we are in alignment, we can continue on. If, however, our experience runs contrary to our objective, we know we are headed *someplace else*. The Alchemist honors native experience as a direct source of information and uses it as one might use radar to inform and direct our journey.

Sounds simple? It *is* that simple! However, as well-conditioned adults we have been trained to doubt our native experience, question our decisions, and worry that we may or may not succeed. It is the unfortunate result of our conditioned learning that has become an impediment to our progress.

I remember when I had started on a newly funded technical engineering program, and business processes were just being developed. Being somewhat inexperienced in finance, I was trying to understand how our budgets were calculated against our progress. I attended many finance meetings and just wasn't able to understand how the calculations were made. I tried and tried, but with little success. Feeling terribly inadequate, I finally mustered up the courage to tell the finance manager that the information just didn't make any sense to me.

I will never forget the finance manager's response: "It doesn't make any sense to me either." Time seemed to stand still as his words echoed in my mind. He didn't understand either! And there I was thinking something was wrong with me all the while.

Over the course of the next couple of days I thought about the incident. I remembered how in grade school I was conditioned to believe that there was only one answer to solving a math problem, that girls were not as good as boys at math, and other falsely manufactured beliefs I had come to believe as a woman working in a man's environment. How wrong I was!

It is unfortunately true, but we all have a backlog of conditioned learning mulling about in our minds that, without the lens of clarity, puts a cork in honoring our native experience. Were we to listen to our radar and honor that native instrumentation, we would question our conditioning. We would assess whether we were going in the right direction, see what was in front of us, and do whatever comes next to head in the direction of our objectives.

We must learn to use the Alchemist's *Instrumentation;* to use our native experience as immediate feedback (radar) about whether to proceed forward or try another approach. If it feels right, keep going. If we need additional information, get it, then keep moving forward. The minute we let our minds take the reins we are likely to end up in The Bog, spending hours rethinking ourselves and changing direction.

I have a bit of imagery that I often use to keep myself on track. I picture a garbage truck to the side of my periphery – I can even hear its loud beeping and see its yellow blinking light. It has a windshield wiper-like arm that can mentally move my worried chatter to the side in a single swoop when I ask it to "clear." I call this the *Debris Wiper!* Then, when I ask myself which of two alternatives seem right and my incessant mental chatter begins to bog me down, I think of the garbage Debris Wiper sweeping my cluttered thoughts to the side, allowing my clear thought to proceed unhindered.

The *Alchemist's Instrument,* then, is a simplifying radar-like tool that honors our native experience as strong feedback, providing the clarifying lens of native feeling that directs us past old, outdated obstacles and towards our Grand Mystery.

The Alchemist Has Two Faces

Have you ever experienced the phenomena where you look into the mirror and think you look great, yet on another day when you look into the mirror you think you look bad? Yet you are looking at the same you! We all have our good days and bad days, times when we are feeling good about ourselves and times when we are experiencing a negative frame of mind. Ups and downs in our own feelings and emotions literally change how we see ourselves. We do, indeed, have two faces.

Once again, the Alchemist has a skill that the novice does not practice – "aware discernment." The practice of "aware discernment" requires two things: 1) the ability to focus attention in the "here and now"; and 2) the ability to distinguish conditioned emotion and mental chatter from native experience.

Remember our second traveler sitting by the side of the trail that we met on the Path of Wellness? He had gotten himself entwined in a flurry of negative thoughts, emotions, and actions. He shared how difficult the path was thus far, complaining about how poorly the trail was kept and saying that he thought the trek wasn't worth the effort. His emotions and thinking were evidence that he was living his life in the "there and then" as opposed to the "now." Perhaps he was experiencing some outdated beliefs that sounded like "life is hard," "don't get dirty," or "cut your losses." We thought he would discontinue his journey on the Path of Wellness and return to where he began – in the pits.

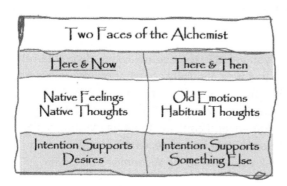

Had he used *aware discernment*, he may have changed his experience entirely. Imagine that as our traveler sat absorbed in discouragement, he tapped into his awareness just enough to admit that he was engaged in negative thought. Using that small bit of awareness, he could then have asked himself, "What do I feel right now?" to which he may have responded, "I am pleased to have stopped for a rest, it feels quite nice." After a few minutes of rest and emotional recovery he may have continued on his train of thought and added, "This rest is giving me some space rethink this experience – I like that."

With those initial thoughts of relief and mild pleasure, our traveler could have begun to reason about the purpose of his initial quest and trail ahead of him. "I really do want to be healthy and I have a very inviting Grand Mystery that calls me; I yearn for that exploration. It is quite rainy out and the trail is very muddy; perhaps I will drape my coat over my head to stay dry. And if my shoes get muddy, does it really matter? This really isn't *that* hard. In fact, it's fun!"

Here our traveler took a moment to reflect on his present moment experience, feel the call of his Grand Mystery, and use lighter language on the *Alchemist's Measure* in order to move into a better-feeling state of mind. In mild increments, we can lighten our heavy load through our words.

It is important to recognize the face with which you are seeing your world. If you are feeling negative emotions, you are assuredly basing your current reality on past experience, prior conditioning. Old emotions have the power to evoke habitual thoughts that will unintentionally reverse your authentic desire such that you are going *"someplace else."*

On the other hand, if you are able to become aware of your current emotions and realize that they are likely conditioned responses from your past habitual thoughts, you can then bring your attention to the "here and now." You can begin to experience your native feelings and thoughts in the moment and continue to move toward the life that you yearn for. Through your language, whether spoken or in thought, you can speak your way up the *Alchemist's Measure.*

We all experience two faces, our "here-and-now" reality and our "then-and-there" existence. The Alchemist, however, uses "aware discernment" to continue the journey through the Quagmire; always returning to the "now" and authentic desire. Grand Mysteries can only be solved in the "world of now." In the "world of then," Grand Mysteries don't even exist.

~

Beside the Lake of Reflection you have learned many things. You have met the Alchemist and it is *you* – you are the Creator of your own life, not the created. Through the power of your thoughts you have the ability, and the responsibility, to create your own future. Life is a never-ending series of "now" moments, with each experience helping you feel your way toward your Grand Mystery. There are no instructions, but isn't that the fun of it?

You have also learned about the Alchemist's three tools: the *Alchemist's Measure,* the *Language of Well-Being,* and your fine-tuned *Instrument* of native feelings and thoughts, emotions, and actions. They are powerful assets and are always helpful in charting your path. With them you can change the course of your life toward vitality, wellness, exhilaration, and love. If you hold a steady pace you will uncover the great *wellspring of unending inspiration.*

As you stand up and stretch beside the lake, you notice that the Path of Wellness quickly brings you to a crossing. There is a sign with two arrows: one arrow looks like a U-turn and directs you to The Bog of Negative Thought. The other arrow, a straight line, points in the direction of The Path of Inspiration.

Next to the sign, the sojourner who danced a pirouette is softly chanting, barely loud enough to hear:

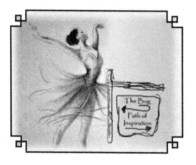

"Dance to the right, learn it with delight!
Struggle to the left, 'someplace else' bereft."

~

Alchemist's Practice

The Alchemist always carries a *toolkit* that helps them reflect on their daily experiences, good and bad, and chart their journey forward based on authentic experience – *"here-and-now" awareness, native feeling and thought,* and *authentic desire* or intention. Through *"aware discernment,"* the Alchemist is always able to travel on the Path of Wellness and live into their inspiration.

The Instrument

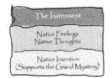

Alchemist's Measure

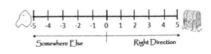

Language of Wellbeing

-4	-3	-2	-1	0	1	2	3	4
Rage / Despondent	Angry / Depressed	Annoyed / Disappointed	Doubt / Frustration	OKAY	Optimism	Pleased	Happy	Love / Appreciation
Grief	Sad	Disappointed	Doubtful	Don't care	Glad	Inspired	Joyful	Ecstatic
Despondent	Depressed	Dissatisfied	Worried	No feelings	Pleased	Satisfied	Confident	Appreciation
Helpless	Angry	Unhappy	Concerned	Okay	Optimistic	Very pleased	Happy	Reverent
Terrified	Frightened	Scared	Frustrated	So-so	Eager	Successful	Strong	Divine
Rage	Rare	Annoyed	Not enough	Fair	Look Forward	Proud	Serene	Love
Hate	Paniced	Missing	Unsettling		Encouraged	Motivated	Calm	Blissful
Impossible		Anxious	Hesitant		Enough	Plenty	Lots	Abundant
					Engaging	Like	Love	In the flow
						Absorbing	Encompasing	

1. Learn to distinguish between the "here and now" and the "then and there." Think about a situation that is causing you negative emotion. Write about the situation, being sure to include what your body feels like, what emotions you are experiencing, and what you are thinking.

_____

_____

_____

_____

2. Reread what you wrote above about your situation in Practice 1, above. Using the *Language of Well-Being* and the *Alchemist's Measure,* make a few notes about the Language you used and the direction you are moving. Add any additional observations you wish to make.

_____

_____

_____

_____

3. Focus on your "here-and-now" experience. Close your eyes and pay attention to how your body feels.

✦ Is it relaxed, tense, achy, calm?

✦ What native feelings and thoughts are you experiencing in the present moment?

✦ If you find yourself drifting into past thinking, bring your attention back to your breath in the present moment. Can you identify what your desire is right now? Do you want to eat, sleep, call a friend, read?

For the next 10 minutes, write about your experience.

_____

_____

_____

_____

_____

_____

Write it down, put words to it.
Compare the 'here and now' with
your 'there and then'. (Practice Often!)

PART II

THE PATH OF INSPIRATION

∞

Chapter 4

~

The Trailhead of Inspiration

Inspiration: a feeling, a desire, Fueling Imagined Future. Feel it—Consciousness Blossoming.

—J. K. S. Zetlan, 2016

The climb up the Path of Wellness was a challenge. Although it was readily tempting to entertain complaint as you ascended the path, repeating the Core Beliefs of the Quagmire kept you grounded and feeling quite positive. The Lake of Reflection has been quite refreshing, too, and you especially love knowing that you could become an Alchemist of Experience and, indeed, craft your inspired life using the Alchemist's tools. They seemed easy to use!

At the crossing, you examine the arrows on the sign. Glancing to the left, toward The Bog of Negative Thought, then to the right, toward the *Path of Inspiration*, you find the choice of direction embarrassingly simple.

"Why would anyone choose to take the path toward the Bog of Negative Thought?" you question, yet you know that you have visited *that place* many times in your life. Definitely the *wrong direction!*

As you look toward the Path of Inspiration there is a landing – *Future's Landing*. You see a wooden bench with a Knapsack leaning up against its side. As you approach it you see that it has your name on it.

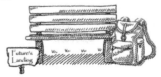

~

Congratulations! You have reached a significant milestone in your journey, and so far it has been a journey of discovery. In Chapter 1, you studied your Grand Mystery and identified the Core Beliefs that will help guide you on your journey. You learned how to challenge those beliefs to enable your personal growth and to open your eyes for the journey, and you established an understanding of the dimensions of wellness (body, mind, spirit, and environment). This knowledge helped set you on your journey and rallied your appreciation that wellness is a conscious choice *made by you*, and provided you a blueprint for how to *live into wellness*.

But we didn't stop there. In the previous chapter we collected the tools to help you continue on your journey to enable you to not only live into wellness, but to *live into inspiration*. These are the Alchemist's tools that remind us that wellness is a choice. We discussed the role of the Alchemist, in each of us, as we build an ever-deepening understanding of human experience and make clear adjustments in ourselves that are in *alignment* with the *futures* that inspire us. We learned that we are the creators of our lives, not the created, and using those tools – the *Measure*, the *Language of Well-Being* and the *Instrument* (our radar) – we can chart a deliberate course forward.

Just as it was important to define wellness before starting your journey, this chapter explores the general nature of inspiration. In addition, we will learn how to clear the "emotional debris" that often blocks our path to inspiration using our familiar Alchemist's tools.

You have come a long way so far along the Path of Wellness. Let's continue that journey on a path less traveled – the *Path of Inspiration.*

Allowing Inspiration

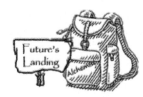

Inspiration is something very different than Wellness. Living into wellness is a choice, but *inspiration is a feeling of desire, an imagined future, that emerges into consciousness spontaneously.* When we live into wellness, we are making choices moment by moment as we respond to feelings, thoughts, and emotions. Inspiration, however, is a native feeling. Our inspiration is ignited when information from Source aligns with desire. It is problem solving at the level of native experience.

A few years ago, my husband and I bought a lovely baby grand piano so he could continue to play his beloved music. To hear him play is like resting my ears in heaven – the complex sounds and melodies seem to transport me magically in space and time. When I asked him how he learned, he would tell me that it was easy; he focused on learning to play chords – in various forms. He then uses that knowledge to create his own personal style by starting with a simply-written melody and adding variations on chords that he had learned. He doesn't play both hands exactly as written, but instead improvises with his knowledge of chords and from experience. Musicians call this "faking," and he owns several "fake-books" to play from.

I, too, had tinkered with playing piano and guitar while in college but found reading notes impossible to memorize and even harder to translate from note into finger movement. It's not that I didn't try! Listening to my husband's music gave me the sensation of playing almost viscerally, but when I sat down to read notes, reality poked a big hole in my desire to play. I never touched our piano because the problem of reading music was difficult for me.

One day while I was struggling to write a chapter I stopped to take a break. I needed relief from my tension, and in a brief moment of silence looked up from the computer and saw the piano. I remembered my husband's description of how he plays. Desire merged with native experience, the visceral feeling gave birth to the inspiration, "I want to play...?" In that moment, I asked him to teach me chords – his starting point – and he paused what he was doing to explain the basics to me. The knowledge "clicked," and I had my starting point.

It was a delicate moment for that inspired idea. The inspiration wasn't a desire with "can't" attached to it. Instead, it was desire and a visceral sensation paired with unmitigated possibility. His approach worked for me! I looked up chords on the Internet – three notes each (triads). I played chords on the right hand, then the left. I still play – it's coming to me, one small desire at a time (like learning "minor chords" next), but now I see the path and follow it one small desire at a time to fulfill my inspiration to play. I am now filled with the possibility of playing beautiful music.

What is this magic of inspiration that suddenly makes the impossible possible? How does the "never before" become a reality? And how do we call on it when we need it?

~

Inspiration is a magical idea. It is what happens in the space of silence without resistance, without our conditioned responses asserting their will. When our interests and needs meet desire, inspiration is born – every time! When resistance is introduced, inspiration is snuffed out like a struggling ember.

The Path of Inspiration is a journey of allowing thoughts and feelings to arise uncensored from within. In the space of silence, of emptiness, native experience has the space to mix with desire and create inspiration. The practiced Alchemist catches the inspiration, nurtures the spark, and keeps its flame alive.

Clearing Debris

Traveling the Path of Inspiration has many challenges. You will often find that the path is filled with debris, challenges large and small that need to be met and cleared aside.

I reflect back on my years in graduate school. I wanted to become a psychotherapist and had to work and go to school to achieve my dream. There were so many trials and tribulations! I was working a full-time job and had to drive an hour from work to school. The schedule was intense and I suffered mononucleosis, an autoimmune disease of exhaustion, because I was overstressed and working so hard to get through my courses. It was a rough two years as I worked, studied for tests, wrote papers, and worried about my grades and my health.

During my internship, I struggled with seeing clients for the first time and had to overcome the obstacles that all new practitioners experience. The phrase "earn your chops" comes to mind.

At times on my educational journey I felt like I was in a sinking canoe, but I bailed out bucket after bucket of water staying afloat. My desire burned strong: I had worked hard to get where I was, and despite mixed emotions, I kept moving forward. Along my path I found a lot of debris that needed to be cleared. The challenge of time, fears of failure, and a little social anxiety often blocked my path. But I tackled them all, one at a time, until my Path of Inspiration was clear – most of the time. That was a good feeling!

On the Path of Inspiration, we learn how to allow inspiration to emerge, how to keep it alive, and how to develop great skill in managing our conditioned feelings. We learn how to clear debris and reduce our own resistance. In this chapter, we are going to learn how to use our bodies, minds, spirits, and environment effectively to ease our journey to inspiration through the Quagmire. Once we develop basic skills, the trek will become a pleasure, a thrill, and an adventure. Once our conditioned thoughts and emotions are tamed

— our nagging resistance — we can keep the flame of desire alive and create our inspired life.

~

As you glance up once again toward the Path of Inspiration you notice there are few travelers. Compared to the Path of Wellness, which was heavily peopled, this is clearly the path less traveled. Your time on the bench at Future's Landing is a decision point. You can pick up your Knapsack with the Alchemist's tools and move forward — or you can return to The Bog of Negative Thought. Your direction is *always* a choice.

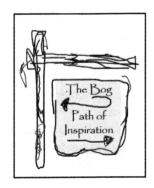

Strategies for the Removal of Debris

Having made the decision to continue on the Path of Inspiration, you will encounter debris along your path. We must learn how to clear the mental or physical flotsam in our path and allow inspiration to emerge naturally.

The Alchemist has tools for this!

To understand which tools to use, it is important to first understand the types of debris you will encounter. There are three types of debris that flourish in the Quagmire:

> ✓ *Deposited Debris* — These are challenges posed by people or situations arising outside ourselves. For example, when you meet a committed pessimist who sees the worst in situations, those pessimistic thoughts become deposited inside you. Hurtful negativity in relationships, as well as office or family politics yields deposited debris. This

deposited debris often results in emotionally charged reactions to others' behavior.

✓ *Habitual Debris* – This type of debris is the habitual or "go-to" reactions to situations that serve no real purpose. Habitual debris can be thought of as over-reactions where kinder, milder behavior would suffice. If you are the committed pessimist offended by another's eternal optimism, you may need to consider removing this interpersonal debris to stay along the path. Sometimes we are the source of our own stumbling!

✓ *Sorrowful Debris* – Often, when pain or grief is overwhelming, we need time to heal our wounds. During these times, we often substitute coping behavior, such as anger, to protect ourselves until we are ready to sort through the deeper issue. Someone who has recently lost a spouse, their health, or a dear companion may display anger, depression, or withdrawal as they struggle to heal internally. Sorrowful debris happens to all of us at one time or another, but when we are ready to manage our loss, we will need to remove the remaining debris before we can fully return to a fully inspired life.

How can we best use the Alchemist's tools to clear the debris along the Path of Inspiration? We are certain to run into it from time to time.

Using a thought experiment to examine strategies for the removal of debris, imagine you are a six-year-old, sitting near a beautiful pond on a sunny day eating an ice cream cone – your favorite flavor. Each lick is better than the last, every moment is perfection. Not too far into lapping up your sweet treat, however, the ice cream topples to the sand, leaving an empty cone in your hand and a sad look on your face. Since you are an Alchemist, you know about native and conditioned feelings and emotions, your spiritual side, your body, and your environment. Based on that knowledge, how would you describe this ice cream experience?

Now consider the same experience, only this time it is another child that knocks the ice cream off its cone.

In a final scenario, consider that another person on the beach knocks your ice cream off its cone, only you are both adults.

Notice how your feelings or emotions shift in each of the scenarios. Tune into what your body might be experiencing as the situation changes.

In the first experiment, it is likely that you felt sad that the ice cream fell to the sand, and as your feelings kicked in perhaps your body reflexively moved to catch the falling treasure ("Oh no!"). As you see the ice cream begin to melt in the sand, perhaps wonder took over as the sweet treat became a thick liquid – fascinating! The next thing you do, being the inspired native six-year-old that you are, is to run back to the vendor with your empty cone to get a replacement scoop. Your hopes are high!

Ah, if only life were so simple.

In the second scenario, another kid on the beach knocks the ice cream out of the cone and onto the sand, leaving you holding an empty cone. Looking at the ice cream in the sand, sadness may have flickered by for a moment, but natively you understood this as an aggressive action as you saw the gallows grin of satisfaction on the other child. That was a scary sight, and you recoiled in fear.

Extending the second scenario, say you came back to the beach a couple of days later, with your fresh new ice cream cone, and once again delighted in the sweet cream. As you look up toward the shoreline, you see the same child that knocked your ice cream over two days ago. You become fearful that the same thing will happen today. The imprint of conditioned emotion and thought has settled into your memory and will be recalled in similar situations; your body tenses in fearful anticipation. The native experience of sadness or wonder at the melting ice cream has been suppressed, as fear has now replaced those conditioned reactions.

In the third scenario, you are now your current age when another adult comes up to you and knocks your ice cream to the ground. You immediately react in anger as you think, "This person really has a chip on his shoulder! He shouldn't be so dumb! You'd think he would know better."

You are now prepared to handle situations like these. You have had many years to learn how to defend yourself from "bullies" and you no longer stand for this type of behavior. In your anger, your blood pressure rises, you pulse speeds up, and your body contracts. You select "fight" over "flight" and let this person know that he should act differently (your words here).

As a budding Alchemist, we practice our debris removal skills by first breaking down situations into their elemental parts, then looking for alternatives that arise from native desire and inspiration.

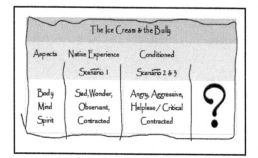

Looking for inspired alternatives in a difficult situation can be hard because we are so familiar with our habitual or painful thinking and emotions. Often, we just react and don't even question them; we believe our reactions are perfectly natural and warranted.

The Alchemist's Tools

By using our Alchemist's tools, however, we can alter the very nature of our thinking and experience to return to our authentically inspired journey. First, we can use *evolved thought* to remove debris caused by the pessimism of others; second, we can go directly to *inspired thought* when habitual debris blocks our path; and finally, we can use *radical compassion* as we begin to heal from deep wounds. Let's take a look at each of the strategies.

Evolved thought requires using the *Alchemist's Measure* and the *Language of Well-Being* to estimate the intensity of your conditioned response, and then using thought and your own internal language to move you toward more moderate thinking. In essence, you are evolving your emotions into greater states of well-being, allowing a gradual return to the inspired experience of your journey.

For *The Ice Cream and the Bully* experiment, let's say that you were going in a direction toward *Someplace Else* at a level -3 and you have been replaying the situation over in your mind creating different versions of "That guy should know better!" with various mental rehearsals of what you will say or do the next time you see him. You know that negative emotion of any size and duration can lead to additional negative thinking, and will move you closer to *Someplace Else* and away from well-being. When you are at that -3 level, a better path will be to feel your way to a better feeling. Perhaps you begin to reason your way up to "annoyed" or simply "concerned." You are going in the *"Right Direction."*

Step by step you can move yourself up through the *Language of Well-Being* to a better-feeling place, and each step in *"the Right Direction"* brings with it a feeling of relief, reducing negative emotions and creating a greater sense of well-being.

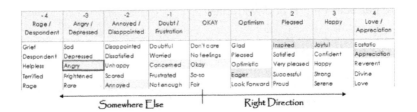

-4 Rage / Despondent	-3 Angry / Depressed	-2 Annoyed / Disappointed	-1 Doubt / Frustration	0 OKAY	1 Optimism	2 Pleased	3 Happy	4 Love / Appreciation
Grief	Sad	Disappointed	Doubtful	Don't care	Glad	Inspired	Joyful	Ecstatic
Despondent	Depressed	Dissatisfied	Worried	No feelings	Pleased	Satisfied	Confident	Appreciation
Helpless	Angry	Unhappy	Concerned	Okay	Optimistic	Very pleased	Happy	Reverent
Terrified	Frightened	Scared	Frustrated	So-so	Eager	Successful	Strong	Divine
Rage	Rare	Annoyed	Not enough	Fair	Look Forward	Proud	Serene	Love

◄——— Somewhere Else | Right Direction ———►

As you get to "OK," take a breather. Pause and notice how far you have come and how the relief from feeling softer has opened up your thinking process. This is a *very important place to rest,* as oftentimes relief meets something new in your native experience and a freshly inspired idea may come to mind. If that happens, stop immediately; take a moment and write it down. Spend time writing something on paper or noting it on your favorite digital "device." You will have just captured an inspired thought! The longer you spend thinking about this inspired idea, the stronger the thought will become and the more likely you are to create a new reality from your thought. You have cleared away the debris in your path!

Inspired thought is the second strategy of debris removal. With *The Ice Cream and the Bully* thought experiment, inspired thought accesses the Alchemist's Instrument by engaging the mental Debris Wiper and moving your own habitual debris, your negative emotion, to the side of your path. Once your debris is swept aside, fresh inspiration is free to emerge. I often imagine this process as visualizing my negative thought being swept to the side of my peripheral vision.

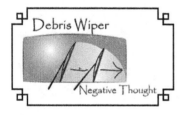

Taking a negative thought and moving it *aside* is an important concept. There is an old adage that says, "What you resist persists." First, resistance – more negative thought – is that piece of debris that falls in your path and blocks your way. Simply acknowledge it, move it to the side of the path, and keep going. It will recede by itself as you move beyond the thought or feeling.

Second, be sure to move the negative emotion or thought to the *side*, keep it mentally on your periphery, but don't try to bury it. Buried emotion burrows within your body and is likely to surface as stress, a cold, or other chronic illness over time. Without being fed additional negative thoughts, it will diminish on its own.

As your negative thought gets moved aside, notice there is nothing ahead in your mental field of vision. This, too, is a relief and is frequently accompanied by a feeling of self-compassion! Simply think about what you *do* want – usually the opposite of what you didn't want in the first place – and note it as your next inspiration. Use the *Language of Well-Being* to move your inspiration to an inspired or joyful place.

Notice how your body feels when you experience relief, self-compassion, and more positive emotions and thoughts. Do you experience less physical tension? Does your chest relax? Does a sigh of relief pass your lips? Draw your *inspired thoughts, feelings, and expanded physical experience* together, as though they were to exist on the same physical plane, or in a symbolic amulet worn close to your heart. They are intricately linked to each other and a resource you can draw upon in the future.

This is the practice of reaching *Inspired Thought*. Daily practice of moving negative thoughts to the side and deliberately allowing inspiration to emerge makes use of the Alchemist's tools. With time and experience you will get much better at moving challenges and other resistant objects to the side of your path, leaving the trail clear for the fresh inspiration that lies before you.

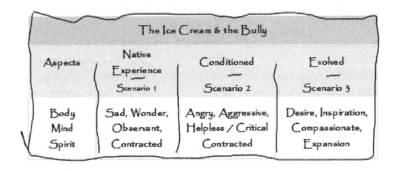

	The Ice Cream & the Bully		
Aspects	Native Experience — Scenario 1	Conditioned — Scenario 2	Evolved — Scenario 3
Body Mind Spirit	Sad, Wonder, Observant, Contracted	Angry, Aggressive, Helpless / Critical Contracted	Desire, Inspiration, Compassionate, Expansion

I worked in large corporations most of my professional life, where politics thrives and the expression of native experience is frowned upon. This is true in many work environments and offers a perfect spot in the Quagmire to practice *inspired thinking*.

In a real life experience I call *The Boss and the Class Act*, a less-than-desirable boss placed me in a position far below my professional abilities. I was enraged (level -4 on the *Alchemist's Measure!*) by the action, but being a single mother at the time, I needed to keep my income stream alive. I could not afford to express my distaste for the experience and needed to adjust quickly.

Without much time to resolve angry emotions and furious thoughts, I promptly engaged the Alchemist's Instrument. It only took a moment to use the Debris Wiper and move my reactive emotions to the side of my path. In the empty space in front of me – what I call *Inspiration's Birthplace* – I posed a Big Question: "What do I want now – in this situation?" It only took a moment for Spirit to present its inspired desire and a new Quest emerged: "I want to enhance this position and do creative work with it – even if it's below my professional level!"

I ventured forth on my new Quest with the passion of any new inspiration, and within the space of a few months had gained recognition and a promotion beyond my original professional role. One manager told me, "You are a class act." It was nice to receive the recognition, but, better yet, I felt ecstatic about the work I did and deeply appreciated that I could live into my inspiration in any situation.

Even after years of experience working with *inspired thought,* there are still times that it needs to be a deliberate response to my challenges. Some situations still hold power over my emotions and behavior, but through evolving my thinking beyond conditioned reactions, and using the Alchemist's tools, I am able to quickly relocate my resistant mind and create the psychic space in front of me for inspiration to arise.

Radical compassion is a highly effective method for removing the sorrowful debris along the Path of Inspiration once you are ready to meet your painful Native Experience. Coping behaviors are protective devices of conditioned thought and emotion we use to help us through difficult times. But, once we are able to identify our thinking as "conditioned," we can choose to go back to the situation that triggered the reaction and trace it back to the earlier Native Experience.

Moving into radical compassion asks us to notice the situation that triggered the conditioned response, and *then* choose self-compassion to replace it. By doing this you can now begin to bypass the conditioned emotion, enabling you to move back into your inspired life.

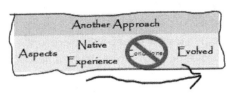

Let's consider a different thought experiment about George and Martha — married for fifteen years. In their seventh year of marriage they began to get into arguments that seemed to start with small issues and escalate quickly into highly volatile screaming matches. The issues that caused a fight varied, but inevitably small arguments would spin out of control, and George and Martha would eventually threaten to leave each other. How would the Alchemist consider this situation?

In this scenario, Martha decides to take some quiet time to reflect on a recent argument. She asks herself, "Why do I get so upset?" and stops to listen to the voice of her native experience. She asks this question several times, each instance getting a different answer when she listens within. Her self-talk exploration went like this?

> *Martha*: "Why do I get so upset?"
> *Deepest self*: George is so inconsiderate!
>
> *Martha*: "But why do I get so upset?"
> *Deepest self*: Because he doesn't listen to me!
>
> *Martha*: "But why do I get so upset?"
> *Deepest self*: Because I hurt inside.
>
> *Martha*: "But why do I get so upset?"
> *Deepest self*: Because my son died seven years ago.

Martha: "But why do I get so upset?"
Deepest self: My pain is still present.

It took Martha about five cycles to repeat her question, but each time she posed it anew it drew her a little closer to her own Native Experience – the premature death of her son.

We often cover our Native Experience with a conditioned thought to relieve our pain. But as we heal, continuously returning to conditioned thought prevents our growth and healing. Returning to Native Experience allows us to begin the healing process. However, when a Native Experience carries with it the burden of pain, we often feel fearful and vulnerable and seek emotional sanctuary wherever we can find it.

Our Spirit, a vital, ever-present resource, is always available within us in the form of self-compassion. With the awareness of a native feeling, we can allow in the nurturing support of Spirit. It may sound like the following:

> *Martha: "How can I ever heal?"*
> *Deepest self: It wasn't your fault.*
>
> *Martha: "How can I ever heal?"*
> *Deepest self: It wasn't your fault, I love you.*
>
> *Martha: Places her hand over her heart and whispers to herself, "It wasn't your fault. I love you."*

Returning to Native Experience and using *radical compassion* to naturally allow inspiration to emerge is a powerful and life-affirming experience. Trust in knowing that there is tremendous dignity in deeply touching your Native Experience and allowing your self-compassion to emerge.

Once we touch the heart of Native Experience, inspiration once again flows forth naturally. Allowing native experience to emerge will always draw self-compassion *and* new inspiration. It is our basic nature and it will never fail.

As a single mother going through divorce I was always concerned that my suffering would negatively affect my son's healthy development. I would sometimes cover up my sadness with overly firm discipline. This bothered me; it was not my desire to parent so unreasonably. As I put myself in "emotional time-out," I traced my behavior back to the Native Experience – existing in the here and now – of unresolved sadness and grief over the divorce. As I experienced the grief, the self-compassionate phrase, "You're doing the best you can!" would arise every time. It brought with it tremendous relief.

In the space of my own self-compassion, new inspiration inevitably arose: taking my son out for yogurt, silly and fun teasing, or other playful behavior. I felt better about *me* and was fully present for my son. I am grateful for the courage and dignity my native experience in the moment provided, and for the playful joy that emerged afterward.

~

Think of situations in your own life that you can reflect upon – in retrospect – and learn to identify the boundaries between *native* feelings and thoughts and *conditioned* emotions and thoughts. This is a powerful boundary to understand, as it gives the Alchemist more clarity about habitual thought patterns and how to discern more beneficial responses. Once you feel comfortable identifying your native versus conditioned experience, begin to use the Alchemist's tools to return your feelings and thoughts toward more inspired choices. Create a quest to move conditioning to the side of your path, re-engage native experience in the here and now, and find inspiration – do what inspires you.

As budding Alchemists, there are tools and strategies we can use to direct ourselves out of The Bog and hasten our journey along the Path of Inspiration. Along the path you will see fewer travelers with conditioned emotions and thoughts, because practicing Alchemists are quick to remove emotional debris and seek out fresh inspiration.

There are times, however, when the Quagmire will present you with other people who pose great challenges. Those are the people whose negative behavior transport you directly back to The Bog.

The Problem with People

People! You've heard the phrase "You can't live with 'em and you can't live without 'em!" Or can you?

Learning to navigate the four aspects of yourself takes deliberation and thought, at least initially, as you gain skill and mastery. As you sit in quiet reflection, or perhaps play with the concepts on a piece of paper, it is possible to get quite proficient at clearing debris with the Alchemist's Tools, returning to Native Experience and moving into evolved or inspired thought and radical compassion. Then, you meet *that person* – it could be anyone – whose unique negativity or different attitude drops you right back into negative thought. Hello Bog.

This is the time to focus on boundaries. The boundary in question with challenging people is to distinguish between "you" and "them." We all live in our own perceptive experience; there is no one absolute version of reality. Each of us has our unique Native Experience, depending on our biology, surroundings, or dominant feeling tones at any given time. Each of us has our personal conditioned history, emotions, and thoughts, and each of us will respond uniquely in any given situation. This knowledge is critical in maintaining your own grounding.

Here's a thought experiment to illustrate. Frankie and Johnny were lovers, but Johnny was raised to believe he was always in the right. Frankie, on the other hand, was not secure in her own native feelings and usually demurred to Johnny's "always right" way of expressing himself. Feeling that she was "not enough," she would take on Johnny's attitudes or beliefs even if they disagreed with her deepest experience of herself. As their relationship progressed, Frankie began to depend on Johnny's view of herself, and his "always right" attitudes began to eat away at her self-esteem. She began to not trust her native feelings, as they rarely agreed with Johnny's "always right" view of her.

One day, Frankie met an astute budding Alchemist, a good friend, who clearly observed their interaction and asked: "Why do you always think your feelings are wrong? You are not Johnny! He *cannot ever* know how you feel."

The trouble with (some) people is they think their version of reality is the only true reality. However, in this varied world that can *never* be true; no two people have identical native experience, identical conditioned thoughts, or identical responses. Therefore, each person lives in their own unique experience and can only depend on their own senses to navigate each path.

If you are Frankie "never right" or Johnny "always right," it is vital that you look to your own experience to chart your way along the Path of Inspiration. We are all in it alone – yet we travel together! It is a beautiful experience to appreciate yourself in the richness of your strengths and weaknesses and another in their own attributes. There is so much to see, so much to learn. Yet we can only remain faithfully loyal to our individual paths, wherever they may lead.

I was raised, as many women are, to trust the opinions of others over my own. I worked throughout my career in a male-dominated engineering environment, where decisive women were not well-received. When I sought mental and emotional safety under the mentorship of a superior I was able to rise quickly in the organization, but after many years felt I had hit the "glass ceiling." I began to understand that my native experience and intellect produced highly valuable results, but I seemed to hit an invisible wall.

As my career progressed I was promoted to higher levels in the organization, until I got to a point where my decisions went peer-to-peer with Johnny "always right" teammates. I found that embracing and holding my native experience and intelligence was the linchpin of leadership. Leadership requires that we remain grounded in native business acumen and stay aligned with what we know to be true in accordance with an industry *and* in alignment with our deeper selves. What I thought was the "glass ceiling" was, in reality, running headlong into a sea of Johnny "always rights." It took years to decipher the key to success with ease. Often I lost the battle in a given role, but, over time, the trust in my own native experience and inspirational alignment helped me win the important wars.

When you meet challenging people along your journey, ground yourself in your own native experience and enjoy the variety of those around you. You *can't* change them, they *can't* change you. Each of you are natively yourselves in feelings, thoughts, and Evolved Thinking. *Vive la différence!* There are many valid and varied approaches to life. Embrace your own and embrace those of others in their differences. Retain your boundaries.

A last word on the problem with (other) people. Johnny "always right" may get disappointed and angry if you do not embrace their version of reality, and Frankie "never right" will blame you if you are wrong. Instead of focusing on their reactions to you, spend your valuable time in this life entertaining your own Frontier Adventure, and support others in theirs. You will find traveling the path together to be a rewarding, growth-promoting, and varied experience.

Freedom

I don't know anyone that does not want freedom from bondage, whether that be from bondage to others or bondage to our own conditioned emotions and thoughts. In fact, the travelers that you will meet on the Path of Inspiration are all seeking that same freedom to uncover their Grand Mysteries.

So, as you begin your journey through the Quagmire – on the Path of Inspiration – spend time learning to remove the conditioned debris along the trail. Each time you stumble on a piece of conditioned emotion or thought, use the *Alchemist's Measure*, the *Language of Well-Being,* or the *Instrument (Debris Wiper)*. Learn the distinctions between *Native* and *Conditioned* experience and feel your way back to living an inspired life.

Work with returning your conditioned experience back into the presence of the here and now. Address your pain with courage and dignity and reap the reward of self-compassion and fresh inspiration.

Practice, practice, practice. In theory, the approach is simple; in reality it can be quite challenging. Learn the boundaries between body, mind, spirit, and environment first. Tackle the boundary challenges posed by other people. The hills to mastery can be steep, but the rewards are great.

~

As you look further down the Path of Inspiration you pause for a rest. You know you have a lot of practice ahead of you and some very difficult people in the Quagmire zap your energy. As you sit beneath the shaded Oak, take the time to marvel in how its roots integrate with the soil and surrounding plants. Revel in how the rain water feeds the earth. Is it possible that how the tree's roots intermingle with its environment holds a message for you?

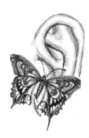

"Yes," says the dancing traveler as she passes you by.

Astonished at this odd coincidence you wonder, *"Did she just read my mind?"*

Alchemist's Practice

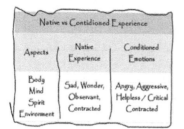

Native vs Contidioned Experience		
Aspects	Native Experience	Conditioned Emotions
Body Mind Spirit Environment	Sad, Wonder, Observant, Contracted	Angry, Aggressive, Helpless / Critical Contracted

Strategies of Debris Removal		
Types of Debris	Available Alchemists Tools	Strategy
Deposited Habitual Sorrowful	Alchemist's Measure Alchemist's Language Debris Wiper	Evolved Thought Inspired Thought Radical Compasson

On the *Path of Inspiration*, you will encounter three types of *debris* — deposited, habitual, and sorrowful. These are conditioned thoughts and emotions, and they make your progress needlessly difficult. The Alchemist learns to identify the type of debris encountered and learns how to use the Alchemist's Tools to clear it. There are three *strategies* to remove debris: Evolved Thought, Inspired Thought, and Radical Compassion. Once debris is removed, inspiration will emerge naturally.

1. Think of a time when someone you know deposited debris along your path: for example, when another person's conditioned emotions affected you. Explore the experience through writing to see what you can learn.

_____

_____

_____

_____

2. Make a list of your own habitual debris: your "go-to" emotional reactions that may be covering your deeper Native Feelings and Thoughts. What Native Feelings did they cover?

Habitual Debris   Cover Up these Native Feelings

_____   _____

_____   _____

_____   _____

_____   _____

3. Describe a time when you encountered your own debris and later discovered that the emotional habit protected you from an experience and feelings you weren't yet ready to resolve.

How would you practice *Radical Compassion?*

_____

_____

_____

_____

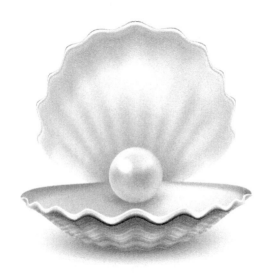

∞

Chapter 5

~

The Meadow of Wholeness

"The one great art is that of making a complete human being of oneself."

–G.I. Gurdjieff

~

"Non-doing simply means letting things be and allowing them to unfold in their own way."

–Jon Kabat-Zinn

Thus far on your Journey through the Quagmire, you are pleased that you have chosen the direction of Wellness and have been practicing how to use the simple, yet powerful, Alchemist's tools to clear the debris of conditioned thought blocking your progress on the Path of Inspiration. Using your Evolved Thought to help you see the world more clearly and with loving compassion – for yourself and others – you are beginning to appreciate your fellow travelers a little more.

"Clearing debris and using Evolved Thought is rather pleasurable," you reflect, "but that odd traveler, the one who dances, is stirring up some uncomfortable feelings – this is terribly unsettling!

"I wish I understood my feelings a little better," you think, "I don't especially like the hard ones!"

You are now ready to look a little deeper into the nature of your Native Feelings and Thoughts.

~

The seeds of your deepest desires and yearnings emerge organically from our native feelings and thoughts. If you experience joy, for example, it may readily evolve into interest or excitement. Alternatively, if you experience anger, hope may appear as your anger diminishes and your desire for something better emerges. Deeply understanding how our native feelings help us actually ensures our survival. They are an important building block for living into inspiration.

Learning about our native feelings and thoughts creates a profound sense of wholeness within us. Once we allow our Native Experience to be felt, we automatically engage authentic desire and inspiration will flow forth. With fewer bottlenecks of conditioned emotion blocking your path, you will begin to see how your body, mind, spirit, and environment work in harmony, perfectly integrated with each other, ensuring that you are going in the *Right Direction* as you seek out your Grand Mystery. This is the experience of *Wholeness*, the integration of all aspects of *you*.

In this chapter, we will explore several innate "feeling patterns" that we all share in common and how they *evolve* smoothly from one into another. As you become familiar with your own unique "feeling patterns," you will discover that they provide a safe harbor for your growth and expansion that will lead you – with deeper trust in yourself – to inspiration. Feeling confident in your own growth process, there is very little that can stop you from joyfully embracing all the challenges of each Quest.

~

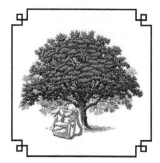

Sitting beneath the strong Oak, you look out over the Meadow of Wholeness, where you will explore the breadth of those "feeling patterns" and learn more about our intrinsic native experience. It's a bit unsettling coming out of the woods of cluttered conditioned thought into the wide-open landscape before you. The soft grasses and low-lying shrubbery lift your heart but give you a slightly disoriented feeling of sprawling emptiness and space. Pausing to adjust, you open your Knapsack and pull out the *Alchemist's Language*.

Surely this tool can help me put words to the feelings I am having!

The Experience of Wholeness

Looking deeply into our own conditioned experience and learning how to return to our native feelings and thoughts can feel a bit unsettling and, at times, scary. Life may have a slightly different quality about it as you come out of a world based on conditioned emotions and thoughts and begin to see the world as it truly is. It can feel confusing and seem as if there are two realities: the one you thought you lived – through your conditioned views of the world – and the one you are living in the present moment – through native experience. As you consider these differences, feelings that we have kept hidden away for years often begin to rise to the surface. This is a short-lived transitional period, and you may feel as if you have two personalities. Rest assured that this is a healthy and normal, albeit uncomfortable, transitional period as we outgrow the myths of our past. We are learning to experience the "now" and how to live into our future.

The first time I experienced the shift between my two worlds – from conditioned to native experience – I had been dating a traveling software engineer. Periodically he would travel from Monday to

Friday, returning on weekends. I was also working hard then, so weeks without my "steady" passed relatively uneventfully.

A project at work was nearing completion, requiring him to be on travel for six consecutive weeks. Being busy with work and childrearing, the first week passed quietly – until the weekend. I had been so busy with work and parenting that I didn't have a lot of activities planned on weekends. I didn't know what to do with my days alone. By the second weekend I was beside myself with loneliness. I can remember lying on my front patio, under the warmth of the sun, crying from fear and loss – six weeks seemed forever!

I cried for a long time, experiencing the burden of feeling alone. When finally I stopped, I poked my head up and looked around the patio. Feeling bewildered, I went for a walk, and, as I did, I noticed the world appeared to have an unusual visual clarity. My feelings of fear and sadness had lifted, like a dark veil being drawn aside, with a bright sunlit day shining before me. I was filled with unrecognizable joy and lightness. As I walked by a small park, I sat on a shallow slope of grass marveling about this unusual shift of consciousness. I didn't understand it, but it felt new and unique; I felt unhampered by sadness or loneliness, simply filled with the freshness of curiosity.

As the next few weeks passed, I experienced a frequent shift in consciousness alternating between the old, familiar feelings of sadness and fear and the uncanny freshness of new eyes on life. In retrospect, I might describe it as undergoing a paradigm shift, a shift of consciousness between my conditioned, anticipated feelings and my native experience, a shift where repeating patterns of thoughts and feelings spontaneously quieted, allowing in a direct experience of my environment.

My alternating shifts of consciousness were unsettling, but intriguing. My conditioned feelings were familiar: I knew how they came and went, but the experience of native feelings was like an endorphin-induced high, a freshness of experience I wanted to stay with me forever! I had made my initial transition from conditioned thinking to native experience!

With time, the range of new feelings became familiar, welcome, and never habitual or negative. They became a highly informative and honest response to life. What were these feelings if not a truly human encounter with both inner and outer life?

In the early 1960s Silvan Tomkins, a Princeton University researcher, studied very young children and the primary effect of feelings, or affect, as the motivating force in human life. He made the assertion that feelings play an evolutionary role in human experience by informing us how to respond to our environment in ways that preserve our species. These primary affects (or, using the Alchemist's language, Native Feelings) are innate and are experienced by all of us:

- Enjoyment, Joy, Ecstasy
- Interest, Excitement
- Surprise, Startle
- Distress, Sadness, Grief, Anguish
- Anxiety, Fear, Terror
- Frustration, Anger, Rage
- Disgust, Contempt, Shame

On the Path of Inspiration, we now come to rest in the Meadow of Wholeness where we observe the sights, sounds, sensations, smells, and tastes of those things around us, as we hope to rediscover our here-and-now native feelings – one by one.

Consider the following scenario – *"Day in the Meadow of Wholeness."*

Sitting under the strong Oak in the Meadow of Wholeness, imagine that you are contemplating how you will rediscover your Native Feelings. You pick up a nearby stone and begin to play with it in your hands. Turning it over in your fingers, feeling its smooth, curved surface, you appreciate its uniquely formed shape. You can discern seven distinct sides – a special stone indeed! A feeling of *joy* sweeps through you as you pass the stone between your hands. It has a comfortable weight as you move it from hand to hand, and you pause in *ecstasy* ("Ah, yes!") as you sit under the Oak, *enjoying* the day. In this moment of joy and ecstasy you are transported into sweet thoughts and images as the urge to play and explore overtakes you. You feel like romping about, expansively, as your imagination and inspiration become shaped by this joy; no thought is unthinkable, nothing is unimaginable.

While you sit in the ecstasy of the moment, you notice the grass before you rustle. Your joy and ecstasy shift gears as your *interest* becomes piqued; you begin to scan the moving grass. A rush of *excitement* floods through your body as you get close enough to see a gentle rabbit nibbling at the grass. You can feel the shiver of goosebumps forming on your skin; your curiosity mounts as you begin to wonder where this animal came from and if there are more nearby. You think, "Wouldn't that be cool!" Interest draws you forward; you want to examine this wonderful creature and explore even more of the meadow.

Wandering deeper into the meadow, you see the grass part before you. Glancing down you see a wet slithering snake weaving its way around your feet. "Whoa!" No amount of joy or excitement could prepare you for this *startling* sight! Reflexively you jump backward to get a safe distance from the winding serpent and almost lose your balance. Feeling a bit *disoriented*, you take a couple of moments to recover your composure and balance to reorient yourself in proximity to the snake. As it continues to slither on its way you are relieved that there is no immediate threat, but it was really good that you reacted as quickly as you did to *evaluate* the situation. It was as if time stood still as you recovered from your momentary disorientation, evaluated the situation, and regained your composure and balance. All other feelings ceased while you reoriented to the Meadow – all that mattered was your safety. Now, with a little more information about the Meadow's wildlife, joy floods back into your body and you resume your interesting and exciting exploration.

Returning to the Oak, you sit back down in its shade and begin to reflect on your day in the Quagmire. Thinking about the rabbit, your mind wanders to the memory of the dog you had as a child. It was a sweet animal that seemed to share your feelings and moods; you felt very close to her, a special bond between nature and you. Sadly, you remember, she was fatally trapped in a kennel fire along with several other families' pets. The *grief* and *sadness,* which still emerge periodically in your heart, make it feel heavy: it hurts, it aches; the *anguish* seems as fresh today as though it were happening right now. Sitting quietly, you allow the feelings to just be. It isn't easy, but, after all, it is a Native Feeling and has emotional importance. With each exhale, you release a little bit of the grief, each breath calming your aching heart.

After a few minutes, as the feelings of sadness begin to melt away, you feel a sense of beauty and appreciation for having had this very sweet relationship – something very unique and cherished in your life; a gift. Picking a nearby daisy, you place it at the base of the tree in sweet remembrance – a memorial for your sweet pup. A gentle sigh escapes your lips as your heart releases its grip.

Glancing across the Meadow you notice that it is getting late, the sun will be setting soon, and you are unprepared for the evening. You are getting cold and hungry, as you think about the encroaching darkness. You haven't yet spent a night alone on your journey without the protection of trees, and there is no firewood nearby to light the darkness. The unknown of the evening looms before you, and *anxiety* begins to take its toll. Your heart races; you swallow hard as you scan the environment for protection, and your mind seems to be scurrying for answers. You hadn't anticipated this, the darkness of night looming just beyond with its *terrors* and surprises! Hoping to ward off the frightening prospects of the night, you look to the sky and petition the universe to keep you safe. You hold up the daisy in ceremonial offering.

As your *anxiety* motivates you to problem solve and find other resources to ensure your safety, you venture out and find a creek with sticks and twigs you can use as kindling. Bringing it back to the Oak, you try to start a fire like a Boy Scout rubbing two sticks together. No luck! *Angry frustration* bursts forth, "Damn rubbing sticks together!" You try again and again until finally, in a near *rage,* you toss the sticks aside. As *terror* sets in, you can feel the agitation bubble up inside your chest, your temples throb in panic, and your blood feels like it going to boil: "I hate this experience and I hate those that talked me into this journey!"

In a cocktail of fear and anger, you stomp down to the creek to see what else may be available to get you through the night. You notice the creek bank has many walnut trees along its edge – dinner! Walking creekside, you gather up as many nuts as you can to store in your Knapsack. It's funny how your fear and anger motivated you to solve the problem of eating! Looking up to the sky again you shout, "But I'm cold!"

Continuing creekside, starting to shiver, you smell fire! At first the smell is startling, but you quickly stop to orient and assess the situation. A small group of people is huddled around a fire, several yards down the creek. Feeling hopeful, you look toward the sky and in relief you utter, "Thank you!" Again you feel your tension drain as you share your relief with the "Great Unknown."

Gently approaching the strangers sitting fireside, you give them a big, enthusiastic greeting. "I thought I was going to freeze in the Meadow tonight – I'm so glad I found you!" With a warm welcome, they invite you to sit by the crackling fire and spend the night in the safety of the group. Since you are in the Meadow beside the Path of Inspiration, it is likely that these are fellow seekers. Scanning the people in the group, you feel safe. "Thank you!" you say to the group, thinking once again that you are saying it to the universe as well.

Within a few minutes of settling in with the group, one of the travelers seems to be dominating the discussion. His attitude is negative, with a bit of a disappointment. He is describing a future dating quest, but his values and attitudes toward his upcoming "conquest" give you a feeling of *disgust* as your body actually cringes as you listen. Tucking you head into your chest you wonder, "How can this person possibly be traveling on the Path of Inspiration?!" The distaste of this person's values and attitudes make your whole body contract; you pick up your Knapsack and move to a spot where it is difficult to make eye contact with him.

With interest, you note that your disgust is a two-part feeling. On the one hand, you feel disgusted and judgmental; but on the other hand, you experience pleasure in knowing your own constructive set of values. You would never want to treat someone as a "conquest," *and* you now know how you might use respect with a future date. Isn't the yin-yang of life interesting! From experiencing something you don't want, you learn what you do want.

As your eyelids start to get heavy with fatigue, you drift into the calm of warmth and companionship.

~

Our Native Feelings are biologically innate and serve us well in our own lives. They support the survival of our species and provide critical environmental feedback guiding us toward healthy, adaptive behavior. Our Native Feelings are short-lived. They quickly recede into memory and always resolve into their opposite – unless they are suppressed, hindered, or only partially released.

The resolution of our feelings always leaves us with the peaceful space of completion and grace. In the space of release and calm, we have created fertile ground for our inspiration to arise. Think about times when your grief eventually resolved into beauty, or the paralysis of fear resolved into action, or anger resolved into compassion, or startle into reorientation. Remember the time when disgust resolved into preference and desire – most likely the driving force behind your Grand Mystery. Take the time to learn and study your own unique patterns of feeling and resolution, paying attention to the end of each feeling – that resolution where the opportunity for inspiration arises.

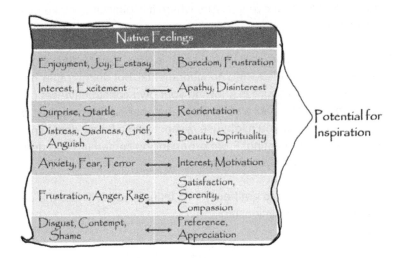

Learning About Our Native Feelings

Our range of possible Native Feelings is vast, yet they form a familiar and dependable internal organization for experiencing our inner lives. Our feelings become familiar, we learn how our unique styles of coping are relatively consistent, and we begin to gain self-confidence in how we process and manage our lives. Recognizing how our patterns of Native Feelings arise and recede will allow us to live in the relative comfort of knowing ourselves.

Sometimes, however, repeating patterns can become limiting. Years ago, I was in a relationship with a "Johnny Always Right." Needing to be right about everything, our conversations would become very one-sided, as I knew it was either his way or the highway. He was often very kind, but his "always right" often got us into disagreements where I would assert my version of reality against his. This became our habitual pattern; our cycle was predictable. We would begin with the joy of being with each other; our romance was always exciting, and we enjoyed each other immensely. But as peak feelings of excitement and intimacy were fulfilled, we would each move into the next area of interest.

My "Johnny Always Right" would often move into desires for his future, such as remodeling his house and landscaping his yard. I, too, would move into desires for my future, which centered on possible marriage and living together. "Johnny Always Right" *knew – for a fact* – that marriage was only a meaningless social construction, yet I thought marriage brought with it greater intimacy and a more meaningful future.

Inevitably, "Johnny Always Right's" opinion of marriage as a "social construction" would stun me as I thought maturing relationships naturally evolved into committed futures. I would experience distress and feel disoriented in the "Johnny Always Right" view of life. How could I ever live in alignment with someone else's view of reality? Anxiety about my own future would arise with the fear and anxiety of being terminally single.

In utter frustration and anger we would argue about our beliefs and our intended futures, and we would eventually end the argument in disgust and contempt over the opposing views of the other. We were each firmly rooted in our unique preferences that these differences brought to the forefront. This was usually followed by not seeing each other for a week or so – until, that is, distance made the heart grow fonder and we would begin to miss each other.

We generally resolved our tension by acknowledging our differences and philosophically appreciating each other's point of view. Neither of us would change our beliefs, but the pleasure of being with each other was undeniable.

In the space of renewed intimacy, we were each making the *choice* to stay together despite our differences and dissatisfactions. We were choosing to live into *conflict and disagreement* (a -2 in the *Language of Well-Being*). We clearly were not going in the *"right direction,"* we were choosing to *"go someplace else."* I began to experience heart palpitations.

Learning how our own internal currents ebb and flow is important in understanding who we are. We learn to experience our Native Feelings, learn about what we do want and what we don't want, and to choose our next direction. Sometimes we choose well, sometimes we don't, and honestly both choices are valid. This is how we evolve and grow; this creates our challenges and supports who we ultimately become. We *always* have the choice to live into well-being or to go someplace else. We also have the choice to change our minds!

When you arrive at a choice point, I highly recommend choosing wellness by allowing your native feelings and thoughts to emerge. Inspiration and adventure are your next step, as long as you choose to go in the *Right Direction* – which is *always* in the direction of your Grand Mystery.

Embracing Transformation and Choice

Periodically in our lives, we feel we need to make big changes. Perhaps we need to change jobs, find a new relationship, or release an unhealthy one. It may be our behavior or lifestyle that is getting in the way of our desired future, but we know that our current trajectory is no longer satisfactory and we desire growth and expansion. When you can feel that encroaching transformation on the horizon, difficult choices need to be made.

Webster's Dictionary would tell you that "transformation" is a change in form or appearance, a metamorphosis in our lifecycle where organic change emerges. In the Alchemist's world, our current state of dissatisfaction will be transmuted into something more desired, more treasured, and more in alignment with our spiritual direction – an *evolution* toward our Grand Mystery.

Transformation begins with the realization of desires and preferences that are rooted in our discontent and judgment. As our discontent peaks, we experience the desire to choose differently. This is the birthplace of inspiration! But what do we choose?

Choice is very simple. For every idea that emerges as a possibility in our minds, there are three options: "I *want* that!"; "I *don't* want that!"; or "I don't have enough information to choose." If you listen in receptive silence to your aware self, one of your innate native experiences will emerge. If the idea brings you joy, interest, excitement, or pleasant surprise – at the organic, native level – that is awareness saying "I want that." If, on the other hand, you innately feel distress, anxiety, frustration, or distaste, awareness is telling you, "I don't want that," Finally, if you feel confused, your awareness is letting you know, "I don't have enough information to choose."

When I was younger and living with my roommate, Amy, we used to play a game we called "Gut Knowing." We were in our late twenties, trying to decide what careers we wanted to pursue. The game began by sitting at the dining room table and writing down a few career choices that we were ruminating about, each on a separate piece of paper. They could be wild dreams or present opportunities (it didn't matter); we just wrote them down and put them in a pile in front of us. After we each created our own pile we would get up to get a snack – an obvious choice at a time like this, often accompanied by a glass of wine. Undoubtedly, we would be making jokes and laughing about our possibilities – this was a game, after all.

We would once again regroup at the dining room table, only this time we traded piles. I had Amy's pile and she had mine. Then, we would go through each idea, one at a time, where we had to express the native feeling to the possible career choice as quickly as possible. We were trying to uncover our deepest desires without the influence of our conditioned emotions and thoughts that seemed to always interfere with desire.

The game would proceed with me holding up one of Amy's cards and reading the career possibility. Amy was required to blurt out her Native Feeling or Thought. Amy's round – she was pursuing an acting career – would go like this:

Career Card	Amy	Action
"Acting school"	"Eew!" (disgust)	Discard
"Dental school"	"I feel like crying!" (sadness/discontent)	Discard
"Get an agent"	"I wish" (interest/desire)	Keep
"Take tomorrow's audition"	Only silence (not enough info)	Research

Amy went on to pursue signing with a theatrical agent. She often had to employ her Debris Wiper to clear her path of conditioned debris that could halt even the most experienced traveler, but it worked and kept her aligned with her Grand Mystery – portraying human experience through acting. Career card by career card, Amy made choices and charted her route on the Path of Inspiration. This particular transformation took her from "Florida Schoolgirl" to "California Actress."

The game sounds simple, almost silly, but it has a very important point. Our Native Feelings and experience are a great resource, and they come to us quickly (if we listen) and provide guidance for our every choice – moment by moment, day by day, or year by year. All it requires is that we stop our internal chatter long enough to listen to our innate feelings, and for the next inspiration or choice to emerge on the way to our Grand Mystery.

What is Wholeness?

As late afternoon fades into to the depth of darkness, you sit creekside with your fellow travelers huddling close to the warm campfire. Knowing what you don't want – to catch the eyes of the negative-minded camper – you realize what you do want. You deeply desire to seek your Grand Mystery in the soothing presence of accepting others, of fellow seekers. It just feels good and there is always something new to discover and explore.

The day in the Meadow of Wholeness has been enlightening. You experienced so many feelings! Joy, ecstasy, interest and excitement – each a natural high, you loved it all. But then there were the difficult times of distress, anxiety, fear, frustration, and downright anger. You even experienced disgust and judgment, feelings you thought you had risen above. You also learned that every feeling has its resolution and that, in the calm of that resolution, inspiration arises spontaneously. What do you call all of these shifting feelings and moods, these moment-by-moment experiences of the greatest variety? You thought living on an even keel was a noble goal, but now you see this is not innately possible.

This is the experience of *Wholeness!* It is living into all that you are in body, mind, spirit and environment, experiencing all that there is to be had in this precious life. But more than living your life fully, it is living your life with *awareness*. That includes the wonder of joy and excitement, the rough waters of sadness and fear, and even the truth of our own conditioning, bad behavior, and outdated habits. We are all that *and* we are the aware observer of all that we are! We are the creators, *not* the created.

Many of us live a richly textured life *without awareness*. It is a conditioned, habitual life, and we don't realize it. We may live with frequently shifting feelings and moods, unaware of their innate value for our growth and survival. It is within our *"unawareness"* that we suffer in repressive thinking or in self-judgment and shame with no apparent exit. Many of us spend our days wrestling with this resistance and living into the lives we *do not want*.

In the Meadow of Wholeness, it is time to relish all that we are – and all that we can become. Embrace your inspiration – what can be imagined is real. Is transformation needed? If it is, take it on – but only in the direction of your Grand Mystery. Does disappointment suggest mid-course correction is needed? Take this as it comes and follow your inspiration.

As your eyelids become heavy in the warmth and comfort of the campfire, your unnerving feelings about the dancing sojourner have thankfully resolved. You remember the seven surfaces of the stone you found beneath the Oak. Your seven types of native feelings! You are indeed lucky to have stopped for the day in the Meadow of Wholeness.

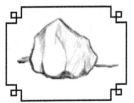

Alchemist's Practice

The experience of *Wholeness* – of living into all that you are in body, mind, spirit, and environment – provides us a lush texture of life experience. Allowing our deeper feelings and emotions to surface can be a challenging experience, but rest assured that the feelings are temporary and will naturally *resolve,* creating a fresh, internal state of quiet. In the *natural resolution of feelings,* there is great potential for inspiration to naturally arise. The Alchemist knows these moments of resolution are rich opportunities.

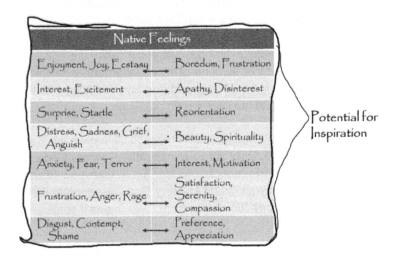

Native Feelings		Potential for Inspiration
Enjoyment, Joy, Ecstasy	→ Boredom, Frustration	
Interest, Excitement	← Apathy, Disinterest	
Surprise, Startle	← Reorientation	
Distress, Sadness, Grief, Anguish	↔ Beauty, Spirituality	
Anxiety, Fear, Terror	← Interest, Motivation	
Frustration, Anger, Rage	→ Satisfaction, Serenity, Compassion	
Disgust, Contempt, Shame	← Preference, Appreciation	

1. Bring yourself into a comfortably seated position on a chair, or on the floor. Closing your eyes, bring your breath into slow and easy inhales and exhales. As you sit quietly, simply notice your thoughts and feelings as they *arise* into consciousness and then *naturally resolve* as they fade into a silent calm.

Take a few minutes to reflect and jot down your own experience. Did you notice a pattern to your feeling state and its resolution?

_____

_____

_____

_____

_____

∞

Chapter 6

~

The Alchemist and the Golem

In the undertow of thought,
Beneath branches of emotion,
Lives mythology. Disguised,
Encroaching, Nipping at our heels.
"I see you." Now and forever
You are gone!

–J. K. S. Zetlan, 2016

~

Don't push the river It flows by itself.

–Fritz Perls

Dawn in the Meadow of Wholeness brings with it the clarity of a good night's sleep and the stunning contrast of early morning sunlight. It is nice to feel the distinct aspects of yourself — body, mind, spirit, and environment — merge harmoniously into a full sense of personal wholeness. This feels powerful — and it is.

Your travels have taught you the value of affirming Core Beliefs, gaining knowledge about the variety of your internal and external experiences and the "feeling/resolution" nature of your Native Feelings. The Alchemist's tools, now stowed in your Knapsack, serve you well in giving you direction, perspective, and focus as you continue to explore your Grand Mysteries. Best of all, you have learned that you can access powerful inspiration in the silence of the mind and internal emptiness. Possibilities flourish.

Packing up your overnight belongings, you bid a heartfelt goodbye to your fellow sojourners and set out once again on the Path of Inspiration. Knowing that you are the creator of your life (not the created) fills you with anticipation of all that lies before you. You continue on into the freshness of morning.

Feeling this greater sense of wholeness, you notice there is a bounce to your step, a lightness in your heart, and a sense of being carefree without the burden of your conditioned baggage. It begins with a little hop, then a step, then another hop...a step...hop...step...skip! You are skipping on the Path of Inspiration and it is exhilarating.

How long have you been skipping? The shrubbery and sparkling, diamond-like stones along the path seem to glide by endlessly as you playfully skip...hop...step. Life is light, you are light, and the future is bright. With a brief jolt of delighted inspiration, you come to a sudden halt, surreptitiously look around – so no one else on the path can see you – and try a little jig. Right toe to the front, then to the back, then a hop. Now the left foot. Again, another try...and another.

Turns out, the jig was not as easy as you imagined – *that traveler sure made dancing look easy!* – and the weight of the Knapsack is just a bit too much. "Oh well," you think, "skipping is good!" and you return to skipping along the Path of Inspiration.

The Wellspring of Inspiration

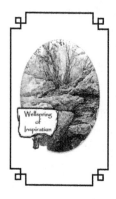

You must have been skipping, on and off, for a very long time, because you are beginning to feel the drawdown of your energy. Pausing beside the trail to refuel with some nuts and apples, you hear a bubbling noise and notice an outcropping of lush greenery. A few feet off the path is a small sign, and beside it a bubbling spring of water defying gravity as it bubbles to the ground's surface and spreads across nearby greens. The sign reads, "Wellspring of Inspiration": a perfect spot for a snack!

Each taste of nut and apple seems to feed your inspiration. As your mind wanders you can see, hear, smell, feel, and taste the essence of your Grand Mystery. Each encounter is filled with joy, interest, and the anxiety of challenge, some quests productive, others perhaps not; always learning as you go. With the use of your Alchemist's skills, there appears no end in sight to all you can experience.

In the distance, you see a fellow traveler – it has been quite a while since you have seen one. As this traveler approaches you wonder why he is coming from your apparent destination, as though he is returning from a quest. Body sunken, head hanging low and slumped he approaches – tears streaming down his mud-splattered face.

You give him the sojourner's sympathetic nod of "hello" as he passes. Stopping when he notices you, he begins to stutter through his tears, "I-I-I can't, I'm dying! It's killing me!" His complexion is pallid and grey; he has scratches along his arms and a spread of mud across him, front and back – a chilling visage before you. "More are coming" he whispers, "No one can stop it!"

Comforting the traveler as best you can, you see others approaching from the same direction; also slumped and withered. They pass by wordlessly. You call to them as they pass, "Where are you going?" One glances back and mutters: "Future's Landing...it's better than The Bog!"

Feeling baffled, and not at all inspired from the experience, you tuck your apples and nuts back into your Knapsack, bid a gentle farewell to the wretched travelers, and make your way forward on the Path of Inspiration. It doesn't take long to remember that their journey is not at all like yours. Fantasies about your Grand Mystery again fill your mind, the imaginative experience coming alive in your body as you take each idea a little deeper into its rich detail.

Until, that is, you notice you are at the bottom of a cliff-like ravine and the only way out is up...or back. (And you are *not* going back!) Looking around, you notice a latticework of interlaced tree roots growing on a twenty-foot vertical sidewall of ravine. With one last look back along the path already traveled, you begin the climb. It is difficult, but you continue to ascend. As you scale the sidewall step by arduous step, doubt floods your body. You are close to the top of the wall, your fingers wrapped around a rock mound on a landing above. As you prepare for that final step onto the landing, where you can start finishing your climb, something clutches at your ankle. You are so close to the top! The traveler's words come back to you: "I can't, I'm dying! It's killing me!"

Meet the Golem

There are times in everyone's life when we struggle to grow beyond our current aspirations. Perhaps we have worked very hard to meet a goal, and success is resting on the horizon. Just as we begin the home stretch to success a deep-rooted fear materializes from deep inside, grasping at our ankles and threatening to pull us into the unknown – the abyss. There is no external threat. What is this experience?

I was a hardworking young adult. I held down a full-time job while completing my post-graduate work and was excited about my upcoming graduation. I had just finished writing the last of my comprehensive exams and was soon to be launched into my much-desired profession. I only had one thing left to do to put that diploma in my hand – drive the thirty miles from my office to the campus to turn in my last paper.

That afternoon when I left the office to drive to campus, the familiar freeway felt overwhelming. What I experienced was far worse than fear or anxiety; it was outright bloodcurdling terror. Looking out the windshield, the clouds appeared almost black-grey and seemed to penetrate a fear deep beneath my skin. I felt like I was going to die! The only reason I didn't turn back was that I wasn't familiar with that part of town. The only safe thing to do was keep on driving – and so I did, in a cold sweat of terror. This was no anxiety attack; there was something much deeper happening.

At home that evening after dropping off my paper, still feeling the threat of death glaring at me from the windowsill, I sat quietly, trying to understand the source of my feelings. What I uncovered was appalling and difficult to sit with: I was enraged at myself for achieving something so desired! (Max on the Alchemist's Measure!)

I wanted to know what thoughts lay beneath these terrible feelings. Looking for a way to navigate to some form of Evolved Thinking I began to ask myself a Big Question: "Why am I so terrified?" The dialogue between my conditioned thinking and deepest self went like this:

> Me: *"Why am I so terrified?"*
> Conditioned self: I don't know.
>
> Me: *"Why don't you know?"*
> Conditioned self: I'm not allowed to know.
> *(great avoidance!)*
>
> Me: *"Why not?"*
> Conditioned self: Because you're not allowed to
> be successful.
>
> Me: *"Why not?"*
> Conditioned self: Because that's not who you are.
>
> Me: *"...And who am I?"*
> Conditioned self: You are nothing.

That was harsh! I sat back and wondered, "Who wrote that script?" It had no bearing in reality, but the experience was deeply real, and rooted within me.

Developmental psychologists have long explored how we make lifelong decisions about who we are based on early experiences in our nuclear family. Depending upon the messages and memories we received as young children we begin to form our self-concept. From groups of experience, what we might call remembered *scenes* of childhood, we construct a mythology about who we are, and will be, in the world. Our mythologies, or stories, are typically formed around the age of five (long before our physical brains mature) and become unconscious *life templates* that set the stage for how we view ourselves and those around us. Once our mythologies have been formed, we begin to view our lives in ways that fit experience into our life templates. They are durable, deeply ingrained, and define the basis our identity.

Imagine the story of Jeanie, a young woman who experienced life through the emotionally abused lens of her mother Dorothy and abusive father Donald. Early life in her family consisted of Dad verbally berating his wife over the lack of perfection in the household; that persistent failure often fell to Jeanie, who couldn't seem to do anything right. Jeanie was often punished for minor offenses, like wiping down the sink with a dishtowel, and by being told her efforts were "worthless." Fear and anxiety were daily experiences in their household, and Jeanie could often be overheard saying to herself, "You never do anything right!" Whenever she did something well, like making decent grades, her success at home was overlooked.

At some point in her early years, and resulting from many similar scenes, Jeanie decided she was *"worthless."* She always deferred to friends and avoided taking on classroom assignments, or jobs, where she had to perform. As an adult, if Jeanie was faced with an important work assignment she would often perform poorly and declare, "I never do anything right!" and then giggle. This was a sorrowful acknowledgement of her *"worthless"* identity. On a project where she stood the chance of success, she invariably would do something just prior to finishing that would cause the project to fail.

Jeanie, early in her life, had decided she was worthless. Repeated scenes in her early family life consistently taught her that she could never do well, and thus in early life she concluded, "I am worthless." Her "worthless" mythology became the template through which she sorted every aspect of her life. As an adult she gravitated toward experiences that fit her mythology, and as an adult she experienced repeated failures. For Jeanie, if nothing else, her life was predictable.

Personal mythologies are powerful entities, and once they are ingrained as a template for life they resist the extinction – the death of an identity – that must occur if they are to be changed. Our full stock of values, beliefs, emotions, and behaviors has been carefully yet unconsciously constructed around our personal mythologies. We mistake these for our true identity. That's why any new belief or other action that threatens to untie these old mythologies from their moorings sends us the message: "Without my mythology I will not exist." Therefore, we seek experiences that *prove the validity* of our life mythology and ensure our character's survival.

Mythologies can also carry a positive tone such as, "I am always right," or, "I am successful." Success myths *appear* less damaging, yet both positive and negative mythologies require that we spend our lives accepting only information that supports our sense of self, rejecting anything that doesn't fit. For negative mythologies, we selectively block out information that lets us know we are valuable. We reject positive input that does not agree with our diminished sense of self. In positive mythologies, we selectively reject constructive criticism, both hurting ourselves and invalidating those around us.

In the course of practicing therapy, I once had a middle-aged client, Eric, who was a high-paid lawyer in the banking industry. He was recently divorced with two grown children, and was living a very upscale life in Marina del Rey, California. He was proud of the fact that he had become a millionaire, but had always lived with the criticism that he wouldn't listen to anyone but himself. He had several "girlfriends" that seemed to come and go, but he was not at all happy in his life. He once shared with me, "Everything I touch turns to gold, but I am empty inside!"

Eric had a Midas mythology many would wish for ("Everything I touch turns to gold!"), but his mythology eventually resulted in alienating his wife and colleagues through his unwillingness to listen to others.

No firmly held mythology will pay the dividends of an inspired life, but is up to each one of us to wrestle with our singular myth-busting fear – the death of our mythical identity.

When I asked Eric about his deepest mystery, he confided that he would love to know the secrets of nature, and if he could, would like to share his findings with the world. He eventually decided to become a naturalist, but the change uprooted his mythological identity of "Everything I touch turns to gold." He would call me with severe panic attacks, feeling like he was going to die. As we discussed the concept of personal mythologies, he began to understand the "story" he had been continuing to live out and decided to pause, explore his deeper desires, and live into his evolving aspirations. For a while he had to take bold new steps forward as a naturalist, with mythological fears of poverty (the businessman's Golem) frequently nipping at his heels. He found the "Debris Wiper" of unique value as he began to replace outdated beliefs and values (like being a high-income producer) with new values (like being an empathic listener) and began to ask daily, "What's next for me – this instant? What's next for me in my dream of becoming a naturalist?"

It took a couple of years to make the transition from "gold-maker" to "earth-saver," but he went on to be an instructor for *Leave No Trace*, working as a wilderness educator who teaches students how to live in nature without leaving any harmful ecological footprint behind.

Identifying your own mythology can be difficult because it is so deeply rooted in our identity that we rarely think about it – somewhat like a fish not being aware it lives in water. However, if you use the *Language of Well-Being*, you may find several clues. Look for old, familiar *phrases* you use to describe yourself at both high and low moments in your life. Here are a few examples that may resonate with you, or they may bring up something else that seems to be a better fit.

+ "I am worthless"
+ "Everything I do turns to gold"
+ "I'm always wrong"
+ "Don't worry about me, I never get what I want"
+ "I'm a survivor"
+ "Don't be me"
+ "Turns out I'm always right"
+ "I'm such a loser"
+ "Bad things always happen to me"
+ "I'm better off seen and not heard"
+ "I'm invisible"
+ "I always do well"
+ "I am always sick"
+ "Things always work out for me"
+ "Don't be seen"
+ "One way or another I always come out on top"

Scanning the list, you can probably see the deep implications rooted in these mythologies. They can be life-threatening at their worst, though helpful at their best. But if yours is a mythology that you must continuously maintain through life choices which prove the storyline to be true, you become a selective perceiver and rule out considering often-crucial internal and external information – both positive and negative. This is never desirable; it keeps reality just beyond your reach.

With awareness, personal mythologies can be changed at any age
– once you have recognized what your personal mythology is...*and*
you allow yourself to become open to possibility.

During the war in Afghanistan, many veterans returned home with
Post-Traumatic Stress Disorder (PTSD) and, often, a deeply altered
vision of mankind. Mark, a young man in his early thirties, had sought
help after his tour of duty. He was unable to function without self-
medicating with alcohol and was severely depressed. When asked
about how he thought about himself, he clearly stated that he had
died in combat – "I'm the living dead," etc. – and all that he did
built upon that story. He sat indoors for long hours at a time without
engaging in anything with interest, and he would blow up into a
rage if challenged with the notion that he was a hero and life had so
much to offer. If he got a job he inevitably did something to "blow
it up," declaring, "why would I care, I'm already dead!" and then a
gallows-grin of acknowledgement would spread across his face.
He responded to his life as though he were the living dead, and
the results of his mythology confirmed the fact of his unfortunate
emotional demise.

Beginning to explore his wartime mythology, he was asked to give
himself a diagnosis. It didn't take long for Mark to diagnose himself
with "Extreme Disillusionment with Humanity." This diagnosis appears
in no textbook, but rather is a clearly personal self-diagnosis of his
own experience: his depleted sense of self and others...and, sadly,
his state of a "living death" consciousness.

Next, we began to explore what a cure might be for Mark's
difficulties, given that he was the "living dead" experiencing "extreme
disillusionment with reality." It didn't take long for him to arrive at
his personalized treatment plan: restoring his sense of goodness in
humanity by supporting returning victims of war.

At first, Mark didn't know where to begin, but meeting after meeting
produced ideas, exploration, and action. He had uncovered his
Grand Mystery – understanding what makes humanity "fully human"
through his contribution of sharing his learning and personal

research with returning soldiers and others who would benefit. There were many Quests to embark upon, such as interviewing victims, families, and politicians, getting at the right questions to ask, and so on. What was once a death sentence became something to live for... and a lifelong purpose.

This is the work of busting your deepest-held mythology – whether it be tragic, sad, or helpful – and resetting your life from where you feel you are today. This is deep and important internal work, and it may take you some time to fully come to grips with the mythology you are living. But this work produces rewards far beyond what yesterday and today offer. In fact, your work will pay off logarithmically (which is huge, even better than exponentially!), by guiding you to create a stronger, more realistic identity about who you are and what might be possible in pursuing your Grand Mystery.

There are times in our lives when we struggle to grow beyond our current aspirations, but it feels like "things are happening" that are pulling us back into the abyss of the past. There may be no apparent reason for your anxiety or fear, and situations in life may seem to pop up out of nowhere that pull you away from your objective. What is happening when you are hitting the wall?

You have just met the Golem, and it is you! The term Golem, a mythological entity of ancient origin, is often used today as a metaphor for a brainless creature created from the dirt of the earth who serves man under controlled conditions but is *hostile* to him under others. In 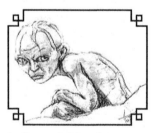 other words, as long as you do not threaten to live outside of your personal mythology, the Golem will work with you to validate your habitual, conditioned self-concept. However, once you begin to chip away at changing your mythology, the Golem gets hostile as he feels *his* impending death.

When working to break out of a non-productive mythology, the feelings of impending doom or death have a mythical reality about them. The death is that of the Golem, the death of a false identity, a false story – of an outdated version of you. This is a wonderful achievement: let it go! Your script is not real; it is a smoke screen covering the authentic, creative, and inspired *you*. You are your clear and ever-present awareness housed in a remarkable physical body; you relish the world's native experience and are the source of joy and creation – *period. Full stop.* There is nothing else.

When dealing with the Golem as it nips at the heels of your progress, recognize that it is a mythical creature from the sands of your past. It is not real; your authentic self is the only reality. Give the Golem a little gratitude for protecting you when you needed him, but then bid him goodbye as you resume your journey.

When I began to do my own myth-busting work, the Golem would nip at my heels at every turn. The night after I faced my Golem, my "you are nothing" myth, I realized that I had a very deep-seated sense of not existing, of being invisible. I decided to become visible. With the encouragement and company of a close friend I went to buy my first new "professional" blouse – not a T-shirt from a hiking trip. I felt the Golem's nip at my ankle – "Don't do this! You are nothing!" – but I bought it anyway. Having had a minor success in buying the blouse, I "inadvertently" tore it on a fence in the first week. There are no accidents; score one for the Golem!

I persisted in busting my lifelong myth by acknowledging a simple truth – "I am someone" – and buying a leather coat. Again, the Golem not only nipped at my heels but tried to pull me down by both ankles, screeching in the caverns of my mind: "You are nothing." The experience was frightening, but with the help of the Debris Wiper and the inspiration to be *someone*, I kept wearing my new jacket and kept it in good condition (I still have it!). Then the next myth-busting challenge came, then another. With further inspiration, persistence, and intention I continued to live into each successive desire – each successive inspiration. Sometimes the Golem nipped at my heels, but when he did I remembered he was only my mythological artifact, moved him to the side of trail, and pursued the next inspiration on the path to being "someone." The more challenges I overcame, the more a meaningful and truthful reality of myself came into place. Next came a new car (I am *someone*), then a job in my professional field (I am *someone* in the field of psychology) and I began to become "*someone* – living an inspired life."

Wrestling with the demon that is defending your personal mythology of the past is a challenge. That is why the Path of Inspiration is the path less traveled. Its voyagers must wage a battle with a fictional entity in a story that may only have seemed real "once upon a time." But once we discern the Golem as being the most insidious mythical creature of the "then and there," we are free to live into our exquisite native experience – the truest reality of all, where we are free to evolve organically, choose a life of wellness and inspiration, and create the lives that we yearn for.

The directions we can choose to travel in the Quagmire are limited. Once you are on the Path of Inspiration and meet the Golem, you can either move that Golem to the sidelines of your journey and resume a richer life filled with inspired ideas, meaning, and possibilities...or you can let the Golem kick you back down into The Bog. It's not a hard choice.

Living into Meaning and Possibility

Gripping the roots on the sidewall of the ravine, one hand on the landing above and the Golem pulling you down by the ankles below, you have an "aha" moment and you realize, "Golems are not real; they are mythical creatures." Memories of the gruesome monster that lived under your bed as a child come to mind: he didn't exist either, and life went on – you could play another day. Focusing on the placement of your hands, you simply pull yourself up another step, and then another, finding footing for each upward gain.

As you crest the top of the ravine, you look back and see no sign of the Golem. As mythically as he appeared, he has vanished into the dirt and mud that formed him. Gazing at the path below and the root wall that you just climbed, you marvel with reflective fascination,

"Wow, *that* was an adventure! *Exactly* what I was hoping for when I started this Quest."

Gazing forward down the Path of Inspiration, then back again into the ravine, you wonder what the experience with the Golem really meant. Was it a challenge, or maybe just a hallucination? Or maybe it was only a very intense childhood memory surfacing in your mind. Searching to find its meaning, you even wonder why it has to have meaning at all.

Humans are "meaning-makers." We all create meanings to thread disparate parts of our lives together as we seek to find value and purpose in the things that we have done. We are also meaning-seekers as we direct ourselves toward activities that promise deeply personal rewards. Meaning is like the glue that fills the gap between past experience and future possibility. Meaning offers continuity of experience from the past to our current state of being in the now, and it creates a bridge to a rewarding and purposeful future.

The separation from my husband after our ten-year marriage brought me powerful meaning in the months following "That Dark Night in August." It meant that a chapter of my life was over, and out of that chapter came a beautiful son, a cherished memory of family, and many remembered years of relative calm. It also meant I had the strength to walk away from abuse (something every woman can do), create personal stability for myself and for my son, and be fully self-sufficient. This was no small achievement!

I had reached the end of one of life's chapters, a plateau of meaning-making where I could put the last ten years of my life in perspective – a mythology, so to speak – and consider the future I hoped to build. It was a period where the past was released and where I bathed in the quiet contemplation of the now. It was a time of imagining possibilities where I could allow desires for the future to organically arise and flourish.

Periodically the Golem tugged at my heels trying to remind me, "You are nothing," but by now I was becoming adept in applying my Debris

Wiper and scuffled it aside, saying, "To dust shall you return!"

Our unique and powerful minds have evolved to create meaning in all that we have experienced. No other individual in modern history has addressed this as insightfully as Viktor Frankl, an Austrian physician who survived many years imprisoned near Dachau during the Holocaust. In a recounting of his experience, Frankl describes how he found deep meaning and purpose to his life during confinement – it kept him alive. He came to conclude that making meaning of life experiences and evolving purpose from them is one of man's primary motivations. In fact, it is *the one thing* we can never lose.

Meaning-making often happens to us in moments of reflection when we ask ourselves, "Why did so-and-so happen to me?" "What purpose did that serve?" or, "What have I learned?" We search for meaning and innovate into our futures. We *create* our life's purpose for which we are intended. This is a deeply personal experience, and when we find meaning, it's as if possibility opens doors before us and calls us to enter.

It is undeniable, though, that as you look back on the experience of the Golem in the ravine, it feels like you have just completed a very important life event – and you have! The demons and myths that held you back last week have been put at bay. Pausing momentarily, you privately thank the Golem for the experience and appreciate that without it you may have never overcome your defining myth – like others, you might have turned back. It has become clear that your encounter with the Golem served to strengthen your resolve, helped you find a deeper meaning in your life, and opened you to new possibilities along the journey to your Grand Mystery.

With possibility on the horizon, you notice that the grey skies have cleared; you can smell the freshness in the air and feel the clarity of your thoughts, and even your vision seems to have become crisper and clearer. The path before you seems filled with curious anticipation. Envisioning your Grand Mystery, and the contributions you will make, you viscerally feel its power and know their purpose in your life.

Through meaning-making we are living examples of our own growth and expansion. In the yoga classes I instruct, after students have challenged their bodies, faced their physical and mental limitations, and touched the spiritual, I conclude with a brief prayer of the heart:

With hands to heart center,
For all you have been;
For all that you are today;
And for all that you will become
In all your tomorrows.
Namaste.

At no other times have I found a group of people sitting in shared experience become as deeply reverent as during this brief interlude. It resonates; it is real. It acknowledges past experience and gives the present meaning; it begs our future possibility and calls us forward — toward all that we can become, toward our Grand Mystery.

It is here, in personal silence, reflection, and meaningful appreciation, that we thank our maker.

We may have held on to long-past mythologies of our earlier years, but we are not trying to preplan a new and improved story. There is an old quip: "Man plans; God laughs!" But it is important to understand how we individually *evolve* and *expand* into the possibilities that shape our futures.

Like the new growth on a plant as it emerges from within itself forming a new bloom, we grow out from the center of our experience, create fresh meaning, possibility, and intention from old growth, and then evolve more fully into our lives. As leaves that have reached their maturity yield to new growth, we too grow beyond yesterday's incarnation and emerge with fresh inspiration, expressing a vulnerable young bud of creation that will gently open to the world. This is how we grow organically, come into new experience, give it meaning, and then expand ourselves to innovate another day. From our prior experience, and from the meaning we have given it, we live into new possibility; we grow organically from the inside out.

It is essential that we learn and actually feel our growth. We must embrace our own possibility and learn to trust our inner guidance. This is as important as learning that the Golem is *mythical.* Our growth is *real,* it has physiological, visual, and visceral qualities about it – it has a purpose.

What if we could keep our eye on our Grand Mystery and, as our internal guidance aligns to it, select the next step that calls us forward. What if you trusted your own awareness and followed your inspiration each step along the journey? This is organic growth emerging out of today's knowledge – not from aged and fallen leaves, yesterday's knowledge, or last decade's memories. Like the plants along our journey, we grow from the inside out. We grow into the lives we yearn for, one meaning, one possibility, and/or one step at a time. We are always evolving – there is an abundance of inspiration, and our journey is never done.

Flow and the River of Experience

Keeping our eye on our Grand Mystery can be an elusive experience. Some days we feel focused, other days we are too busy with the "stuff" of our lives, and sometimes our minds simply wander as though we were floating along aimlessly.

The metaphor of a river is a good way to view our lives from a longer-term perspective. As we know, a river flows in one direction – what we think of as downstream – and is filled with any number of obstacles. Sometimes we can see these dangers, but at other times we are unaware of them because they rest below the water's surface. If we imagine ourselves in a relatively quiet section of river where there are no obstacles above or below the water, we have the sensation of being "in the flow" with the water and its environment. Our ride is comfortable, the banks of the river pass gently by, and we feel ease and contentment as we flow with nature in its natural rhythms.

Continuing to float downstream, imagine an outcropping of boulders and fallen branches ahead of you. If you are looking ahead, most likely you have time to navigate around the obstacles and the journey is one of manageable challenge. However, if we are too tired to pay attention, or become otherwise distracted, by the time we see the obstacles we will need to switch into crisis mode to avoid collision.

Sometimes we get hung up on an obstacle, like the outcropping of a branch – or someone's opinion – and we try to navigate upstream to get free of it. Paddling upstream is exhausting; maybe you will fix the situation, maybe you won't, and surely the effort has taken you out of the natural flow of the river's current. It won't take long to realize swimming upstream is no fun, and overall produces few results.

So it is with our journey through the Quagmire. Understanding the pull toward our Grand Mystery and "knowing" the value of our eventual contribution – our treasure – it is possible to flow in the current of our uniquely created lives without trying to get ahead of ourselves, swimming upstream, or getting distracted.

Finding your individual flow in the river of life calls on you to hone your perceptions and awareness; you must trust in Native Experience to guide your direction. But how do you recognize "flow?"

There are a number of physical, mental, spiritual, and environmental clues that are always signaling to you about your "flow status." But first, you must learn what flow feels like to know if you are in it or if you are providing resistance.

To recognize flow, picture yourself floating down a meandering river. The current is smooth and allows you to feel safe and stable, even as your raft gently rocks amid the current. Sensing inside your body, you feel the slow release of your muscles, the feeling of internal spaciousness as your blood circulates freely, nourishing your heart, lungs, and other organs. Looking downriver and towards the river's banks, you see only smooth waters – the shoreline sands and greenery flow past at a mesmerizing rate. The sounds of birds and the gentle breeze compliment your feelings. The sun's warmth cradles you in movement as the river carries you downstream.

Try now to apply this metaphor to your life. Notice how, at times, the pace of your life has a comfortable ease about it. You have the time to relax naturally into the day's events, and there are no opposing forces or abrupt disturbances. You likely experience a sense of calm and tranquility; your muscles are somewhat relaxed, and the flow of energy within your body circulates evenly with each breath. Your heartbeat feels slow and regular, and your stomach is quiet and relaxed; you feel a sense of competence and focus. Notice how events in your life seem to arise, often at just the right time. The pacing of your life seems to strike a balance between the outer world and your inner experience. Often it feels like you can see into your past: the present and the direction, or "vector," of your future – simultaneously. Look inward at how your awareness is perfectly aligned with intention, thought, and action. This is the experience of flow.

Naturally, we run into obstacles. Undercurrents may tow us temporarily downward, and some situations pose challenges and upsets, but all-in-all there appears to be a progressive sequencing to your life. The more we align ourselves with our Grand Mystery and our deeply personal intentions, the more conflict-free life becomes, no matter what difficulties we encounter. Our challenge is to navigate the currents of our lives, both external and internal, by choosing those paths that clearly forward our progress.

Once we allow distractions to derail our direction, we introduce *resistance* toward uncovering our Grand Mystery and reaching our treasure; we begin to swim upstream. We may shrink ourselves in the face of inspired choices, push against another's opinion, or fight against a feeling of our own that we find uncomfortable. Some clues to resistance, or swimming upstream, are a quickening of the heart, the feeling of tension in your neck, shoulders, or back – your stomach may feel clenched, or you may feel frustrated or upset. The more energy we devote to our distractions – self-doubt, fear, or worry – the more we swim against the current of our own intentions.

We begin to feel exhausted, exasperated, and discouraged. Our inner and outer worlds feel mismatched; we are so busy managing distraction that we lose sight of our own Grand Mystery, native feelings, and sense of meaningful direction. Life loses its native pleasure – inspiration stops.

In order to evolve and grow into our expanded selves – to organically *live into inspiration* – we must allow ourselves to recognize and orient ourselves to the flow within our lives. When we get into our own flow, life comes to us as we can manage it; our bodies, mind, and spirit are alert and we execute life confidently and effectively. Even if difficult circumstances come to us unexpectedly, we are able to restabilize quickly in Native Experience and focus clearly on "what's next." When we are in the flow of our own life – in alignment with our Grand Mystery and our treasure – we are able to grow and evolve organically.

We must set up an early warning system to recognize distractions. Without a sensitivity to our inner experience, life's events will cause unnecessary stress and tension and lead to imbalances in health, emotions, relationships, and self-care. Practice honing your awareness to detect subtle emotional and physical indicators or resistance, and resist swimming upstream in pursuit of distraction. Notice when resistance starts, and what you do to stop it; become familiar with your own inner currents of flow, distraction, and resistance.

Finally, practice returning yourself from a state of tension and resistance back to your natural flow. (It is always easier to begin practicing with easy problems.) The clues of resistance are in your body with aches and tension, they are in your mind through scattered and negative thinking, they show themselves spiritually when you feel disconnected and isolated, and they show environmentally when the spaces around you reflect your disarray.

Actively seek out your internal clues of flow: physical well-being (muscular ease, slow and easy breath, a sense of pleasurable energy, pleasant sleepiness), appreciation of Native Experience, feelings of connection and love, and a satisfying, nurturing environment (even in the presence of chaos).

Learn to quickly "right" yourself into life's flow. Sit quietly and seat yourself in the native experience happening all around you. Ask yourself, "What is the experience of my now?" (name it in this moment), find the rhythm of your own breath, and consciously breathe into your abdomen and chest – no matter what's happening around you. Stop, look, and gently ask yourself, "What's next?" and listen to your answer. You might surprise yourself!

Whenever I find myself swimming upstream I am reminded of the quote from Fritz Perls,

> *"Don't push the river, it flows by itself."*

Evolving into the Future

Learning to clear the debris out of your way as you travel toward your Grand Mystery brings with it new feelings of freedom – in our hearts and our minds, our spirit draws in the world and relishes in fresh possibility and inspiration. We want more, and we learn that with the use of the Alchemist's tools we can have it whenever we wish. It is nice to fully comprehend that we are the creators of our life, not created by some external force. We set out on our journey with a skip in our step, ready for whatever comes next.

Just when we think we are well on our way to living an inspired life, we often encounter a part of ourselves we weren't quite aware of – the story of our lives, an actual mythology about who we think we are that was authored in our early childhood experiences. Our mythologies can frame ourselves as pitiful victims, grand kings or queens, or perishable humans as we continually go through life, proving the truth of our stories. Our Golem would even fight to the death to defend them.

We now know that our mythologies, and our Golem, are not real. They are fictions drawn from the scenes of childhood and crafted together by the children we once were. We created our stories through the eyes of babes, not through the hearts and minds of grown adults. However, as adults, we can understand that the myths and the Golem are imaginary vestiges of our ancient history.

Once you come face to face with the Golem, you have found a perfect time to use the Debris Wiper and compassionately tuck our old identities away in a corner of our Knapsack. We would never want to forget these, as they are the chrysalises that shaped us. They held the seeds of our Grand Mysteries; yet once they are understood, we are obligated to tuck them away – if we are to thrive.

Our chrysalis holds a very personal meaning for each of us that awaits our discovery. As we emerge from its fable, our lives begin to take on fresh perspective. Our Grand Mystery begins to unfold before us in a more meaningful way, and our contributions, our treasured offerings, take on the deep, rich glow of value and purpose in our emerging lives.

We glance ahead at the terrain that lies before us, and possibility lights up our path. Moment by moment, day by day, and year by year, we continue to emerge and evolve into all that we will become.

~

Several yards away, as the Path of Inspiration curves slightly to the left, you see an enormous, naturally shaded tree root that spreads horizontally along the side of the trail. Possibility shimmies across your mindscape as you create an imaginal "Bench of Reflection" out of what, moments ago, was simply a tree root. What a perfect spot to rest as you reflect upon all that this Path has brought to you, your insights from the Golem, and the anticipation of what lies ahead on your way to your Grand Mystery.

You do a quick little dance, take off your boots, then lay down on the bench for a short nap.

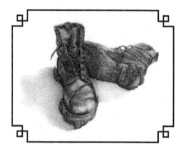

Alchemist's Practice

Each of us has a deeply rooted *mythology* that establishes our subtle inner identity and sets the stage for future decision-making about ourselves. These mythologies can be negative in nature, or they can feel positive, but they are all fictions of our past. Our mythologies are born out of childhood events and parental messages and laced together into a story by our young and inexperienced minds. We rarely think about them – unless we are attempting to go against the script. That is when be become aware of our *Golem* – an often scary experience. However, if you use the Language of Well-Being, you may find several clues.

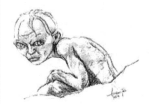

Clues that the Golem is Nipping at Your Heels

- I am worthless
- Everything I do turns to gold
- I'm always wrong
- I'm a survivor
- Don't be me
- I'm invisible
- I am always sick
- Things always work out for me

✦ "I am worthless"

✦ "Everything I do turns to gold"

✦ "I'm always wrong"

✦ "I'm a survivor"

✦ "Don't be me"

✦ "I'm invisible"

✦ "I am always sick"

✦ "Things always work out for me"

1. Using the *Alchemist's Language*, look for old, familiar *phrases* you use to describe yourself at both high and low moments in your life. List them here.

---

2. Describe how you would use the Alchemist's Tools to remove the Golem's debris.

_____

_____

_____

_____

_____

PART III

LEARNING TO DANCE

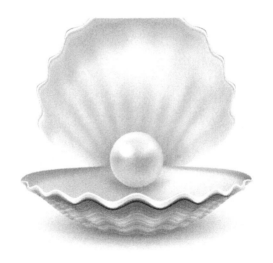

∞

Chapter 7

~

Learning the Steps

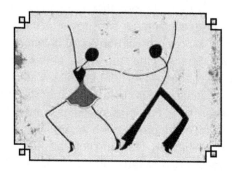

*"Stop looking all over the place for "the answers"
– whatever they are –and start looking for
the questions – the inquiries which are most
important in your life, and give them answers.
You do not live each day to discover what it
holds for you, but to create it [each day anew]."*

–Neale Donald Walsch

There is nothing better than waking up from a good rest!

From the Bench of Reflection, as you gaze first in front of you, then to
each side, you see a myriad of narrow paths weaving in and around
a secret garden. (There is a sign nearby that reads, "The Secret

Garden.") Leaves edge the paths in sweeping, curvy lines, with fragrant bouquets folding into, then rising above bright shrubbery. The landscape is so pristine that you wonder whether landscapers created this paradise, but you know that it is so deep into the Quagmire, only the garden's travelers could have made this so.

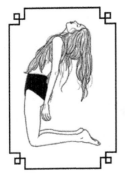 To the right on the path nearest you is the traveler, the dancer, skipping like you had done on the Path of Inspiration. You look for the familiar hop...skip...hop, but she seems to be doing something different. It is as though she was repeating a few distinct steps over and over again. First, she would step forwards on her right foot, then bring forward her left while reaching her arms towards the sky. Holding the pose, she struggles for balance – the ground looks very uneven. She tries the step again, better this time; then better the next. Next, she follows her bent elbow as she turns to the right, carefully negotiating a full circle. Stopping, she looks very pleased with herself. Next, her arms stretch upward as if pleading with the heavens, then she draws her hands down softly and lays them gently across her heart. Now she links all three moves together, and again she looks very pleased. Suddenly, she kneels on the ground, tilting her head up toward the sky and stays there, swaying as if enraptured. She holds the pose for several seconds.

Finally, she stands up with both arms outstretched to her sides, turning right and then left – as though she were surveying everything around her. At last she returns to a standstill and seems to bow a *Namaste*. She repeats the same movement sequence over and over for a very long time.

This is not skipping; this appears to be the steps of a dance, carefully sequenced and repeated over and over until each movement flows smoothly, perfectly, into one another until it looks easy and natural.

"Are you dancing?" you ask as you try to catch her during a moment of stillness.

"This is the *Dance of Inspiration*. I have been learning to master it for quite some time," she gladly answers. "It's very hard to go further into the Quagmire unless you can dance with inspiration, so I am practicing until I can do it easily. My Grand Mystery calls loudly, and I know that this is the next step in my travels."

Thanking her, and offering gratitude for her candid answer, you return to the tree root, your "Bench of Reflection," to give this answer some thought. What does dancing have to with a Grand Mystery? On the other hand, you did try a jig on the Path of Inspiration.

Dancing is not something that comes easily to you, but neither was traveling the Path of Wellness – and you did that – and you have surely overcome your Golem!

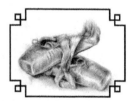

Dancing into Inspiration

Sitting on the Bench of Reflection, an obvious question arises: "What do I dance to?" Getting up to ask the dancer what music she is dancing to, you notice she has completely disappeared. In her place is a sign that reads, "*The Alchemist's Garden*." You are certain it wasn't here before, but on the other hand, you hadn't asked the question about dancing either. Feeling obliged to return to your inspired journey, you begin to feel a bit irritated, "I don't have time for a puzzle! I *need* to keep going!"

We all wish we could live lives seeking that which inspires us rather than being pulled relentlessly forward by obligation. In other words, we have a deep-rooted desire to live and act in alignment with our true self within the flow of our own lives calling us toward our Grand Mystery. However, for the vast majority of us, we must work to provide enough income to support ourselves, our families, and our lifestyles; or we must provide the emotional and domestic support to our families that enables everyone to thrive. We do what we have to do, or what we *should* do, to get by or get ahead. When we have a dream, we tend to put if off – not for long (we tell ourselves) – into a gauzy future where the practical demands on our lives will surely have become less pressing. This is a part of Humanity's Myth that we weave into our mythologies: "When my children are grown...," "When I have the money...," "When I retire...," "When I win the lotto...," and so on.

In the meantime, we pinch off our inspiration and continue to build constricted lives so we may, at a minimum, maintain the status quo. We look at our lives today and plan for the immediate future, say tomorrow or next month, and decide what needs to be done. We keep an arm's distance from our dreams so we may maintain what we have today; we perpetuate our busy and stressful lifestyles; we live out Humanity's Myth.

This is living from the "outside in," living to meet our mounting obligations. We live into today and figure out how to patch through to tomorrow. Our inspiration (our dreams, our passions, and our joy) is put on hold.

How, then, do we shift gears so we may live an inspired life? We *know* it is possible, we feel it in our gut, in our hearts. We can feel a low-grade wellspring of diffused desire that whispers to us quietly from a deep sense of spirit. We have an idea what will make us feel joy, but words and thoughts don't help us achieve clarity of purpose.

We have learned that an inspired life is built upon the expansion of our ever-evolving self as we grow and seek to fulfill our dreams. There *is* an abundance of energy and well-being all around us, but the channels for expression feel vague or unclear. Somehow, we must learn to flow with the river of our life and learn when to use the anchors that ground us with love, safety, familiarity, and comfort.

Each of our anchors – people, relationships, pursuits, goals, or anything else that you cherish and love in your heart – is a living wellspring of inspiration, growing and changing as we walk our path. (We'll learn more about these "seedling anchors" in Chapter 8, when we enter the Alchemist's Garden.) Let's pause and look at how inspiration actually enters our hearts and our minds, and consider how we can nourish its emergence.

The Mystery of Inspiration

I have to thank my mother for raising me on the phrase "Do what inspires you." There is an obvious truth to the idea, but putting it into practice can be a lifelong pursuit. Left to our own devices and our everyday stresses, life constantly provides us with distractions that leave us feeling as though we are "living into a fractured life." This happens when you realize that "I want *this*, but I'm doing *that*." Let's look a little deeper, in slow motion, at the birth of inspiration (a snapshot in time, as it were), to understand where inspiration originates. If we can understand how it arises, we can learn to harness the process and "ignite" it as we wish. Remember, we are the creators, not the created!

Inspiration is the birth of an idea as it sparks from seeming nothingness; a yen, a desire that arises in our minds from our sense perceptions. We all get ideas, we all have sparks of creativity that fire up randomly in thought, but to live an inspired life we must first learn to recognize inspiration when it arises and then learn how to harness its presence and persistence.

Have you ever experienced a jolting idea? Perhaps in surprise you thought, "Wow, that idea came to me out of the *blue!*" Inspiration can be felt as an actual sensation that is sometimes described as a tiny electrical jolt in your body, where your sensory neurons literally receive and transmit the environment's charge of energy, and the body releases a cocktail of pleasurable chemicals such as endorphins or serotonin. The spark of your sensory neurons then trigger others along a dense chain of neurons in thousands of areas in your brain, channeling impulses from to the memory banks deep within the limbic system of your brain. It is searching for recognition – for a feeling that has been previously stored. Your mid-brain begins to add information to the sensation (the Who, When, Where, and How of the memory), and your cortex (the uppermost layer of your brain) finds the language and concepts that would translate the experience into structured thought and language. The origin of an idea can be very subtle or quite pronounced, depending on how much you allow yourself to open to the world around you and how receptive you are to experiencing these feelings, impulses, and thoughts inside of your own body.

In this next thought experiment, "The Sound of One Train Passing," let's slow down time and look carefully at how inspiration forms. Imagine the following: You are sitting in a quiet room on the second story of a building. The window is open, and a warm calming breeze brushes over your skin in a most pleasing way. You are appreciating the feeling of the gentle air and relishing a moment of absolute quiet. Outside your room, there is a lovely, tree-lined neighborhood with a small commuter train line twenty-five yards away. The streets are somewhat narrow, flanked with tall buildings; any sounds or vibrations that might ricochet through these little canyons are sure to be amplified. As you sit in peaceful repose, you notice the sound of the commuter train coming. At exactly what point do you hear the sound of the distant crossing signal begin to clang? As the train nears and crosses the closest line of your perception you are fully aware of the train, but when does the sound of the train diminish into nothingness?

The elegance of this simple scenario demonstrates how an idea is quietly sparked in your mind. The environment around you sets the preconditions of your perceptions. In "The Sound of One Train Passing," you are relaxed and sitting in a peaceful and pleasing room; your senses are not being bombarded by external noise or motion. The environment outside of your room is also pleasing, and as a result, you are feeling safe and at ease. In short, you are experiencing a mindful state of consciousness and your sensory organs are in a receptive state. As you rest in mindfulness, your senses are awake and registering changes in sound, vibration, or other environmental inputs. The approaching train reaches the distance where it begins to be barely perceptible to your ears, depending on your sensitivity to sound – your eardrums register the crossing signal's vibration. Do you experience delight at the faint clanging sound? Or does it give you an annoying uncomfortable sensation?

Observing your process closely, you would notice that your mind now begins to search your memory banks looking to translate the experience of the vibration into a feeling, concept, or word that you are familiar with. Perhaps this is a familiar vibration, and as the vibration continues to resonate over the next few milliseconds, you sort through your experience and match this sound vibration to the concept of a train crossing signal. You have *translated* a vibration into a word.

Imagine another case, then, where you had neither ever seen a train nor experienced crossing signals. You would experience the vibration and search your memory banks for a reasonable translation, but you would come up with nothing to classify this unfamiliar event with. To account for the experience, you would either have to make up a word, or ask another person whether they had ever heard such a thing. Your mind would puzzle at the experience until somehow you could find or create a translation of the experience that you might store away for future reference.

Interestingly, a characteristic of our neurophysiology is that we remain on alert with our problem-solving thinking until we mentally connect a perception to a word or concept. This is the experience of ruminating on a problem until a solution appears. We *need* such closure when we experience something outside of our experience.

Inspiration, then, can be thought of as the point at which you receive subtle (or not so subtle) vibration from your environment and translate this vibration, or energy, into a native experience (which might or might not feel good). Next, the feeling calls forth a thought that suggests a next action to resolve the circuit. Depending on whether the experience felt good or not, you will either want to approach the idea or get away from it. And from that experience, inspiration – *the spark to act* – is born.

This slow-motion explanation of inspiration is important to understand as we engage environment and spirit and *allow* them to work together to infuse us with inspiration. Environmental stimuli within us and outside of us merge and invite us into action. The translation of the spark into action is the *divine mystery* of perception, a mid-brain translation of experience that is uniquely our own. Ideas are wonderful creations offered up by the world around us and within us, and from the moment of inception we become creators of our own world. *We* have the experience, *we* spark an inspiration, and *we* create whatever comes next.

Leading an Inspired Life

We all live inspired lives, whether we are aware of it or not. One would hope we were inspired for the good, but simply watching the news tells us, "That just ain't so." We look at politics in the world, or in our work or home environments, and recognize that people are inspired to do both good and bad things. It is here that we need to literally "consider the source."

Any inspiration that initiates directly from source (or environment) and is joined with our unique native experience (our spirit) is a divine expression of the partnership between our world, the universe, and ourselves. It is an act of translation: from perception, to desire, and then into inspired action. Native inspiration can be trusted; it is innately true; it is the result of direct personal experience and is *always* aligned with the world around us.

However, any inspiration that gets filtered through our conditioned thoughts and emotions is, by definition, distorted. All experience is first sensed, then translated...but conditioned emotions then get translated a *second* time into something that has been through the mental and emotional filters of our past. This *recycled inspiration* is filtered through our own conditioned mythologies: it's like a second-generation inspiration. It is always out of alignment with our true selves, since it has gone through a second translation. Thus, we can be inspired to seek revenge, inflict hurt, or grab power – all examples

174

of *second-generation recycled inspiration*. Steer clear of these inspirations, because they will never get you what you truly want.

It is true inspiration – alignment to our native inner selves – that we seek. These moments of inspiration are always in synchrony with nature, and they flow naturally in the river of our lives. They feel good, and we want more of them. The Zen Buddhists use the term "Tao" – translated as "the Way" – to describe how the world flows around us and within us. We are part of our moving stream of objects, perception, and consciousness. Both our minds and our environments are ever changing, moment by moment. We are magnificent receptors of our worlds, and we can choose to move about with the ebb and flow of the "Tao," or push against it. When we allow ourselves to live in the flow of the now we feel glorious, at one with all that is. When we push against nature's way we feel discord and we suffer.

Fritz Perls, a Gestalt psychotherapist in the 1960s, once said, "Don't push the river, it flows by itself," meaning that life has a natural way of unfolding before us and with us, we should relax and enjoy the ride. It is exactly this experience we want to achieve through living into inspiration. This is how living an *inspired life* begins – allowing your inspiration to arise, being mindful that each inspiration is in alignment with the deep nature of your life, and that any aligned inspiration is a worthy endeavor. Constricting native inspiration is a step *toward someplace else, cutting off life's natural flow.*

When I first graduated college with a degree in behavioral sciences, I sought out a position working with developmentally disabled children in special programs. As I spent time providing therapy to the children, I noticed there were several adults with disabilities not receiving speech and language therapy. I felt it was very unfair to ignore the needs of the adults as they, too, could benefit from learning to talk and get their basic needs met.

At the time, I was working with an agency that I felt could have implemented its programs for adults but was choosing not to do so. I remember my first day at work, opening the double doors of a sheltered workshop for adults and feeling the spark of inspiration galvanize in my mind. All at once I knew what was needed, and I was deeply inspired to provide services to them. Both they and their families could benefit greatly, and it would thrill me to explore this area of my profession. I continued to grow dissatisfied with my organization – I wanted to grow into my inspiration but my agency was not receptive to the idea. It became clear to me that I did not want to stay in a static practice, and I desired to expand deeper into a field where I might accomplish things that had yet be tried.

During that time, a friend of mine suggested I call the local Regional Center to see if there were other programs that served adults – perhaps I could get a more satisfying job. The Center referred me to a speech pathologist, Shel, and he and I struck up a passionate conversation about the adult population. We decided, on the spot, to start up our own agency with developmentally disabled adults and their families.

We began to build the company a week later. All the pieces of the business puzzle fell into place. Acting on one inspiration after another we met people that were eager to support and fund us, clients who welcomed us, and families that needed our help. We found the flow within our environment and within ourselves and paddled downstream effortlessly. Within a few years, we had built a clientele of over four hundred and fifty clients; our group of therapists was made up of committed, mission-driven professionals, and the company created a new space and methodology in the treatment of developmentally disabled adults.

Without being aware of my own process of inspiration, yet with no resistance or worries with regard to building a new business startup, I rode the wave of inspiration. I was on the cutting edge of my own thinking and forged new pathways in the industry. I stayed focused and did not get distracted by opinions saying "You can't" or "Don't," and there were many of these. My strong inspiration, combined with the flow of the industry, my partner Shel, and a clear vision, created an unstoppable force – distraction be damned!

In retrospect, I can see how the power of inspiration – my refusal to be distracted by any resistance – opened up new pathways in the world. I was living a grand adventure as I traversed the paths and ravines toward my Grand Mystery...uncovering the nature of "mankind." I flowed smoothly for ten years, as I stayed in tune with my native inspiration and honored the flow of life's currents.

I had many similar experiences of alignment, of riding my inner inspirations and honoring the awareness of life's flow. I began to test the process: *Perception + native inspiration + action = flow*, one step at a time. There was a very clear alchemy of inspiration in operation.

There was period of time when, as a project manager, my program was near the close of a contract and I needed to find another job. I searched inside myself for the next inspiration and came up blank. No ideas; the well was dry.

It was then that I decided to put the *process of inspiration* to test. As I experienced myself in the "now," I came up blank, so I decided to fully embrace my *"blank-ness"* and honor that native feeling and experience. I remembered the Cheshire Cat's phrase from *Alice in Wonderland:* "If you don't know where you're going, any road will get you there." So I decided to take a pause in life's journey and simply explore the nearby paths to see what might be next for me. This was a very vague and formless idea, and I did not create any specific plans for exploration. I metaphorically hopped into the flow of life's current and shared my inspiration to embrace the "blankness" and desire to explore with my friends. I set out to test the universe and the process of inspiration.

As I embraced the "blankness," as I rafted in the flow of life's current with the intention to explore, it was as if possibilities of exciting adventures came directly into to my mental inbox. Job interviews started coming in, and I began to examine which career possibilities seemed like the most *fun* – which jobs piqued my interest, which offered adventure, and which might offer me opportunities for the greatest personal expansion. I pushed the envelope of each job interview to see what might be possible (my translation: *fun for me*) until the final candidate rose to the top of list.

I accepted my next job (my new Frontier Adventure) in the Bay Area, relocated my son and me, and never looked back.

This *process of inspiration* is something every Alchemist must learn. It is available to all of us, every moment of every day. It's there for the asking; all we need to do is to *allow* ourselves the opportunity for mindfulness (a quiet focus on perception and feeling), to *value* our native inspiration by embellishing and nurturing its persistence, and *hop into the current* of life's flow.

The Process of Inspiration

How do we harness our inspiration? We all have great ideas and desires that waft briefly across our minds but, being the well-conditioned people that we are, tend to dismiss these ideas with well-worn phrases such as "Yes but...," "Yeah, well," or some other brief act of dismissal. We tend to look at the reality around us and think, "That could never work," and then continue to live our lives in the same manner that we told ourselves moments before that we didn't like. Perhaps we listen to those around us – our boss, coworkers, friends, partner, etc. – and back away from our ideas, being discouraged by negative input or thinking that others see something we don't. Let's take a look at the *Process of Inspiration* and get a better understanding of the *value* of our sparked ideas.

If we look at the *Process of Inspiration* at a very high level, we could summarize it quite simply:

1. *Esteem Yourself:* Rest in the knowledge that *"we are"* (we exist in nature), *"we are a given"* and *"we get to pick"* our future. No action needed.

2. *Become Quiet:* Empty your mind, and allow mindful awareness to create perceptual and emotional *space.* Empty the vessel.

3. *Ask Important Questions:* Explore. *"Who am I?" "What are my anchors?" "What do I want?" "And what comes next?"* Then listen to your own answers.

4. *Marinate:* Allow the thoughts to root and grow. Always do what's next.

5. *Look:* For evidence of success.

Esteem Yourself

We have come into this life and have accumulated decades of knowledge, experience, successes, lessons learned, wisdom, and understanding. We each have a unique history, we each perceive things from our own broader experience and perspective, and no one has information about our lives to the present day, or what should come next, better than we do. No one! Simply put, "We are." We ourselves get to select each new step in our unique and personal Frontier Adventure.

We all, at times, look back at our lives and see our successes and our failures. We also tend to spend significantly more time on the things that are not pleasing, are disappointing, or are missing than we do on those things that are positive and complete. These are not the ruminations of a negative-minded person, but a natural *"feature"* of the yin and yang of existence.

Our frustrating habit of focusing on the negatives rather than the positives was first discovered by a psychologist named Bluma Zeigarnik at the University of Berlin in 1927. She was at dinner with her professor, Gestalt psychologist Kurt Lewin, and noticed that their waiter had strong recollections of still-unpaid orders but forgot the details of orders that had already been paid. Bluma decided to design a series of experiments to uncover why this was so. She gave test subjects a list of sentences that were a mixture of complete and incomplete sentences and found that most recalled the incomplete items while forgetting those sentences which were fully complete. With these results, and other similar studies, Bluma concluded that incomplete events establish a sustained tension that awaits resolution. This phenomenon has come be known as the Zeigarnik Effect.

We can recognize this mental behavior in ourselves when we ruminate over a problem that has not yet been resolved. We seek closure, or resolution of the issue, so we may find relief from the tension-causing thought and go on to other activities. Thus, when we notice repetitive thinking or behaviors in ourselves, rest assured our brains are performing as intended. *We are perfect* just the way we are. From our need for closure, inspiration calls to us from the horizon; our inspiration invites us to expand and grow further.

Another valuable attribute we humans possess, and must become master artists at, is the ability to both act and react. If we were able to live without the influence of conditioning, or learned behaviors and thoughts, we would act and evolve quite naturally. We would expand our lives and grow with our natural capabilities with ease. We would know that our emotions and instincts are valuable tools. We would never "push the river" – we would naturally flow with it, doing what comes next through awareness and choice. We would trust our instincts and listen to our gut feelings. We wouldn't feel shame or embarrassment from being who we are deep inside. We would just be.

However, we are culturally trained to constrict the flow of our inspiration, to do as we are taught, and to contain the natural ebb and flow of our emotions. We find ourselves "overcoming" our "weaknesses," at times by brute willfulness. What if we could stop and make a choice to identify our native desire and *act into the next moment,* then choose to act into the next moment, and so on. We would begin to act instead of react; flow naturally into our tomorrows, not patch our way into them. We would begin to thrive.

As you rest in a calm moment, know that you were made perfectly for *you.* You are a precisely crafted human who has the gift to know what is good for you and what is not. No one else has your unique biology, history, experience, and feelings. You are nature's work in progress, designed to expand and grow into the future that you desire – without end. You are able to discern what is going well and what remains to be done. You are able to act with grace into a life that you love.

Become Quiet and Allow Mindfulness

Most people find sitting quietly a difficult task. Our minds are constantly generating thoughts, and there seems to be no end to our internal chatter. This is our natural mental machinery in constant operation, and it can feel impossible to control. In the world of yoga, a practitioner will strenuously exercise their body and mind for one to two hours before being ready to take the traditional pose of Savasana – the most difficult of all yogic postures. In Savasana, one lies flat on the ground with legs and arms extended. The instruction for this pose is to relax, bring your attention to your breath, and allow your thoughts to come and go naturally, without grasping onto any one of them. Simply allow your thoughts to emerge into your field of awareness, and exit with the breath. You would be surprised at the number of people who cannot remain still for five minutes without squirming, shifting position, and even getting up to move about.

Yet, it is this very familiarity with stillness that we need to cultivate in order to move through our thought machinery, our incomplete memories, worries, myths, or reminders of things to do. Those thoughts tend to clutter our minds and distract us from experiencing the now. "Know Thyself." How can we possibly know ourselves, if we can't quiet ourselves long enough to experience our true centered self – that part of us that communes with the world around us and translates the vibrations of perception into information and inspiration.

Several years ago, after relocating to the Bay Area, I was feeling upset over a new friendship. My friend planned a trip to the area and didn't have time to visit me; I was feeling angry and ignored. I didn't like feeling that bad over a relatively small issue and tried to soothe myself. I was in my upstairs den and asked myself, "How am I feeling *right now?*" Very simple observations came immediately to mind: I felt cozy wrapped up in my blanket. My den was on the second story of my home; surrounded by trees outside the window, I felt like a bird resting safely in my treehouse nest. Looking around, I noticed the angles of the room, which were not all perpendicular, and the two-tone paint on the walls, which was quite beautiful and artistic. I then noticed how comfortable and pleased I was, in general, to be in this lovely room, feeling so cozy and complete. In that second I noticed my joy at being me, in my den *at that moment.* It was a lovely experience, and I discovered a simple technique that I use frequently to feel comfortable and at peace.

If we follow history back to the earliest mystical writings, we see the human body referred to as a vessel. Even mind was described as an empty vessel awaiting the mixture of experience, feeling, and thought to create an idea, a concept, an inspiration. We each have our own mystical alchemy coming together every day. The products of this mystical alchemy become thoughts, thoughts become actions, and actions become things. It is a perfect system – until we constrict ourselves or let our Golem stop us.

Our vessel *can* be constricted, with challenging consequences. If our machinery gets clogged by the ceaseless cacophony of our minds, if our channels of native perception and feeling are cut off or replaced by the myths of conditioned living – then we begin to create thoughts, behaviors, or objects that cannot flow freely in the river of life. Our thoughts and feelings become distorted and our reactions are not native outcomes of what we perceive. We experience the sensation of resistance, of a pushing against our own idea, or another person's thought or opinion. We feel like we are straining to swim upstream against the current. We are pushing the river.

Allow yourself to become quiet, to empty the body/mind vessel and deeply experience the phenomenon of *you* in the *now.* Become the observer – the witness to all that you are – and know that you are perfect. No exceptions.

Ask, and Then Listen – Part I

Neale Donald Walsch, author of the 1995 international bestselling book *Conversations with God*, wrote a series of books documenting conversations with his inner self. His practice was to simply ask god a question and listen for the response. Answers to his own questions came from what one might call spirit, inner self, our observer, or god. It doesn't matter which word you choose; however, we all have the ability to connect deeply within ourselves to find our perceiver of reality. We have direct perceptual connection to the world around us, and our observer (or "inner self") is our vibrational translator and trusted advisor.

We all have access to the wisdom and understanding of our deepest self. All we need to do is *ask* a question and then *listen*. If we listen, we will hear – we seek resolution to our question. (Remember Bluma and the distracted waiter!) Our own inner voice always provides answers, direction, and insight based on our native perceptions. Our inner source can be trusted. *Always*.

As you continue to sit quietly and "empty the vessel," pose a question to your inner you. Perhaps you ask if you should have salad or chicken for dinner, or perhaps you ask if you should take "this" job or "that." Then just quiet your mind and listen – your inner voice *will* answer.

Before I moved to the Bay Area, I was interviewing for jobs. Two positions rose to the top of the interview heap: one inside my current company, another in a different company. Both jobs were exciting, yet very different from each other. I did the logical exercise of creating lists, pro and con, for each company, talking to friends and family, but nothing helped. I still couldn't decide. I crafted a simple question to ask my inner self: "Which job should I take?" I asked the question, then listened for the answer.

My inner voice spoke immediately, but not with a quick "this" or "that" answer. It simply said "There's not enough information yet to decide. Just let things evolve, you don't need to do anything...*[don't push the river...]*," I thought, "Wow, that feels true, why didn't I think of that?"

As the days passed, I waited "for things to evolve." As it turned out, one of the interviewers from the external company had a change of heart about the position, and my original company said they needed me immediately, offered me a generous relocation package, and found me corporate housing. My inner voice ("There's not enough information yet to decide. Just let things evolve...") had given me sound guidance. Sometimes in life there are moments so unique, so unusually profound, that they imprint in memory. This experience was one of them. It was one of those rare experiences where you discover a miracle about the mysterious way the universe operates.

I encourage you to test the validity of your inner voice. Ask important questions, and then listen closely to your inner advisor for the answer. You will consistently find profound results! The questions come easily, but learning to listen to your inner voice's answer takes some practice. Don't get discouraged, just ask, empty the vessel, and *listen*.

Ask, and Then Listen – Part II

There is a Part II for "Ask, and Then Listen." Here, we go deeper with your questioning. As far back as mankind has been recorded, philosophers and scholars have asked the question, "Why am I here?" or, "Who am I?" This is a central question that we all, at one time or another, wrestle with. This is a perfect time to *Ask, and Then Listen.* The answer is there, you have a deep inner knowing – you just have to empty the vessel, ask the question, and listen.

I was once in a business meeting where several people had volunteered to support the development of the ideas in a research essay on the subject of "Asking, Then Listening." I asked each advisor to describe how their spiritual DNA, their core inner self, could be described. The team sat in quiet, more from the strangeness of the question than from anything else. Slowly, one person after another began to speak. One man described himself as simply an "uplifter": "I uplift people; I want people in my life to have positive experiences." Another person commented she was a "border collie," always making sure everyone was well, doing what they wanted or needed, and had their needs met. "I always know deep inside where everyone is and that they are OK. I can't sleep at night until I know everyone is alright." The answers to this central question about your own DNA will have an uncanny sameness over time, yet it is possible that elements of them change over time, depending on the situation.

There is a second question to be asked. It is not enough to simply ask, "Who am I?" It's informative, but of no use unless applied to living into your inspiration. The next question to ask is, "What comes next?" Quiet your mind, empty the vessel, and then listen once again.

Karen, a young woman in leadership I had been coaching in the dominantly male-dominated high tech world, shared with me that there were no readily available women role models she could emulate or learn from. She knew several other women who, like herself, were searching for women in leadership but seeming to find only slim pickings. I suggested she ask herself, "Who am I (as a woman in the high tech world)?" and "What is my mission?" I hoped her own answer would lead her to her own identity, her personal leadership DNA.

Some days later after Karen asked her question, she shared with me that her inner voice was silent for a long time, as if holding court on her behalf. Then finally on her drive home from work her inner self responded to the question and told her, *"You* are a leader. There are no role models, *you* are the role model."

Karen's own answer seemed to ground her in a new identity based on the environment around her – she was indeed one of the more mature and experienced women in the densely male-populated organization and, if not her, who else could serve as a role model for other aspiring women? The answer came to her clearly, but if felt daunting.

As she was telling me her story, a George Carlin quote came to mind: "Always do what's next." Although the question seemed humorous, it was spot on.

So I asked Karen: "OK, if you are the role model, then what's next?"

Her answer: "Hold myself in esteem as a leader."

Karen's description of her inner voice came through loud and clear; I could see her posture change. She sat more upright, literally "holding" herself in esteem, and her expression altered from "worrisome little girl" to "confident professional." Even her energy changed; she appeared somehow bigger, she became a larger version of herself with purpose and direction.

Even though this experience happened many years ago, Karen still holds that core sense of being a role model in her career. She related to me that her inner voice taught her to act in the absence of direction, to trust her native knowledge in the face of the unknown, and to stay aligned to her mission of providing a role model for others.

We are all magnificent humans with abilities and powers we are yet to really understand through the scientific method. But we have them; the ancients spoke about them in *The Book of Creation*, *The Yoga Sutras*, and in other historic and well-known scholarly writings. We have so many resources at our fingertips, we need only to seek, experiment, and honor the results. We are more than our physical bodies and our constrained minds. We have our connection to the greater world around us, and within us, of vibration, inspiration, and creation.

Marinate, Then Act – Allow Inspiration to Take Root and Grow

As we consider the important questions in our life, ask for guidance from our inner selves, and listen to the voice of spirit, inspiration spontaneously emerges into our mindscapes. Inspiration is the spark that has been born within us. It is a mixture of all that we have ever been, the sum total of our experience, all that we know and all that we perceive. It is a perfect mix of perception, feelings, and thoughts as they present themselves. Inspiration takes a new shape in the moment the question is asked. Embrace the question, listen to your inner guidance, and then seize the thought. Catch hold of the inspirational idea and *nurture* it. Use the powers of your focused mind to think, imagine, envision, and speak your inspiration. The more time you spend thinking about what inspires you, the more your idea will mature, grow, and come to life. Let your inspiration marinate, allow your imagination to embellish the idea, play it out in your mind, do research, ask more questions, and add more detail to your vision. The bottom line is to embrace the embryonic thought and allow it to take root, evolve, and expand.

Years ago, I formulated a question that I knew I would keep me on the edge of inspiration for years to come. Having been in the corporate world my entire adult life, I wanted a change where I might have more ability to impact the world in the coming decades. I started to review the story of my life. I looked at my life as though someone I just met (and presumably after a couple of drinks) asked me, "What's your story?"

I began to write a brief story of my life where I recounted my experience as a young child losing my father to an early heart attack, my years in college and my ten-year long internship as a psychotherapist, my marriages, my kids, and so on. I wrote about my highs and my lows, my strengths, and my challenges. It wasn't a fancy story, but it was an honest accounting and a loving "look back" at who I have been.

After I completed the story, I reviewed it to see if anything of interest popped out that might inform my life today. It was inspiring to take a bird's-eye view of my life. I noticed that the "character-building" incidents in my life began to follow consistent themes. There were issues about spirituality and world concerns that drew a lot of passionate interest. The threads and maturation through each of life's decades, or phases, seemed to form an earthy progression as my values and beliefs were formed and strengthened, or others disproved. I became curious about me in the "now," and how I might harness my talents and desires over the next several decades.

As I reflected and saw the threads of inspiration sprout and grow throughout my life, I crafted the next question: "What would thrill me and keep me on the edge of my own personal adventure through to my nineties?" I had a Grand Mystery, but I was unsure of my mode of contribution. In other words, "What is my life's mission, my Quest?"

What emerged in the final paragraph of my Life's Story was an articulated mission, or Quest, for my future: "My Quest is to bring a deeper sense of spirituality into the world – for practical people." It wasn't lengthy, it wasn't fancy, but as I imagined that Quest in each area of my life, new inspiration seemed abundant. I could see bringing a deeper sense of spirituality and connectedness to each of my anchors. I asked more questions: "For my children – how could I deepen their sense of spirituality? In my marriage, how could I deepen the spiritual connection with my husband? In my career, how could I deepen spiritual exploration in my work?" and so on.

And then the sublime happened. I remembered that George Carlin quote: "Always do what's next." I asked the question as it pertained to my life and to each Quest: "Then, what's next?" I picked my career as an area to explore first, and over the next few months a vision began to emerge, steeped in the inspiration of bringing deeper spirituality into my career.

This activity of *asking, listening, and marinating* in the inspiration of my life's Quests began to take root. I frequently reviewed my Grand Mystery with its Quest as it became woven Into my career expansion and kept asking "What's next?" to make my inspiration and ideas a reality. I marinated in each expanding idea – usually over a quiet cup of coffee.

Over the year that followed, I became a certified yoga instructor, transitioned out of the corporate world, started a book, and began lecturing in the Bay Area. I have not looked back since I started the process, and I experience new inspiration every day with each new challenge. Each morning, with my cup of joe, I reflect on my Career Quest and ask the simple question, "What's next?" Returning to this question makes me think over what I might do (whether in career, with family, or with friends) that would be in alignment with my deepest self. Each time I empty the vessel, reflect, and ask an important question, I find myself re-launching into my Frontier Adventure – that place in my life where each next step carries me into an expansion, a bigger version of me with an abundance of inspiration.

Look for Evidence of Success

As you begin to act from inspiration, embracing your alignment with source and your deepest sense of self, look for evidence of progress and forward movement. As you ask, "What's next?" and take each successive step, stay alert to even the smallest accomplishments. It is so easy to take minor accomplishments for granted, but each day's baby steps, or milestones, keep you *living into your inspired life.* Each day spent following and acting in alignment with Source and spirit, with your Quests, you spend *living into inspiration.*

Sometimes we get impatient looking to complete a Quest, or a goal, immediately: today. We want an achievement *now*, we don't want setbacks. We only keep our eyes on the horizon, without appreciating our progress, our commitment, our resilience – or our mental, emotional, and physical well-being. But keep in mind that a mission embraced with clear focus is a life's journey worth having, an experience that takes a lifetime. By the way, you control the pace at which your dreams become realities. More on this later!

Distraction

We have choices about how we live our lives. On the one hand, we can put off today's inspiration for a more conducive time. This means we can choose to move our native experience, feelings, thoughts, and inspiration to the side, as we follow the life we would actually like to change. We can constrict desire, awaiting better timing. On the other hand, we can choose to listen to source and spirit and explore our desires and what truly calls to us in this life.

In the former, we cut ourselves off from our inspiration and true feelings; we choose to live into our mythologies with all their illogical untruths, illusions, and shoulds. It is a choice; we become *fractured* as we live *apart* from our native selves. Or we can listen to our deeper selves and find a way to follow our inspiration. The second approach is much easier on our spiritual, mental, and physical well-being...and is much more rewarding.

First, let's look at an illustration of *fractured living*. We're going to tell a story that we'll call "The Hose" – read below, and try to find the point in time when a decision leads away from leading an inspired life.

Imagine that you love gardening and are on a Quest to raise a magnificent tree. Your tree has thick, rich bark and sturdy branches with large, green, radiant leaves that form a cascading canopy above the grass. You are on your way to nourish it with water from the garden hose. You turn on the water and watch a short spurt of water spray out the nozzle of the hose, but then stop. Thinking the water wasn't strong enough to come out, you double back and give the nozzle another couple of twists. The next thing you hear is a pop, and a stream of water shoots up into the air from a rupture in the hose. A quick panic shoots through your gut. Not being a trained "hose technician," you go into the garage, get some duct tape, and wind a few layers of on top of the puncture. Returning to test the water flow, you turn on the water and the tape holds perfectly.

Then...*pop!* Another stream of water shoots into the air from another spot. Ugh!

Next, you go online to research hose repair and watering technique. This is a little irritating since you have work to do, but it's got to be done. You notice an online gardening site where you can chat with other gardening hobbyists, so you join the discussion group. Over the next week you spend several hours discussing irrigation systems with people online. Some of the people decide to meet at a local nursery to do some gardening research.

The following month, in frustration, you give up trying to repair the hose and call in a landscaper – who, of course, has significant hourly rates – to repair the problem. The landscaper comes in and notices that your hose had a kink in it that caused the flow of water to constrict at the kink, where water pressure would build up until it could puncture the hose wall to release the pressure.

Although it would've been an easy problem to fix if it had been diagnosed at the time the water was constricted ("I should have seen that!"), it was now a problem requiring either a puncture repair or a new hose, each of which involved an outlay of lost time and money.

Where did fractured living begin?

Fractured living began at the duct tape. You were living the dream, following your inspiration until a distraction literally "popped" up. You got distracted by shoring up the hose's *symptoms*. In fact, you got hooked into conducting a Do-It-Yourself repair, but it became a much longer-term distraction since you needed to find a chat room, call in a landscaper, and spend time and money on something secondary to your original inspiration.

Thinking we need to spend our time maintaining today's challenges leads to lost time, lost money, and poorly-spent emotional energy. It usually results in spending *more* time, money, and energy just to get the job done. Before you know it, many hours in the week are being spent in projects out of alignment with your core inspiration. This was not your desire to begin with, but here you are – living a fractured life out of alignment with your initial inspiration.

Perhaps this analogy can be compared to a physical condition my friend Maria experienced. Maria had been working long fifty-hour weeks and was under firm deadlines leading to a product test. To keep her mind off the job stress on the weekends, she filled her days with activities and distractions. After a couple of months Maria began experiencing frequent headaches and stomach tightness, so she made an appointment to see her doctor. Following the physical examination, her doctor diagnosed her with hypertension (frightening!) and prescribed a blood pressure medication. In the weeks that followed, Maria's symptoms came under control, and she resumed her tough schedule and busy weekends. "Problem resolved," thought Maria.

Then, eight months later, at a follow-up exam, Maria's kidney function appeared to be below normal and she was diagnosed with her second chronic ailment ("I'm falling apart!"). Of course, there was a medication for that, although the doctor recommended she significantly change her salt intake. Maria's daily life resumed as usual, but the fact that she was showing signs of chronic illness nagged at the back of her mind. Maria's husband and kids started showing concern for her health, and began asking her to take care of herself. She assured them she was carefully taking her meds as prescribed and that she was doing just fine. This was the year that preceded Maria's heart attack.

Maria's hypertension story is an example of how fractured living can cause you to *live into illness,* and can ultimately pull you off the path of your Grand Mystery. During her recuperation, Maria began to rethink what had happened to her so she could avoid another crisis in the future. She began to think that at the early signs of stress and social over-commitment, instead of powering through at work, she could have decided to take a little downtime and listen to the needs of her body. Looking back, Maria noticed that her busy and overcommitted lifestyle was leading her to experience burnout and fatigue, body signals she chose to ignore and which eventually led to a health crisis. Her health crisis also caused her to lose weeks of work which, unfortunately, impacted her career progression.

Maria committed to living into wellness, something she was now inspired to do. Maria spent time on the weekends to "catch up" on some much needed rest and reflection after her work week. During her weekend downtime, she discovered that her crammed schedule at work was the result of poor planning at the company and she clearly *did not want* to burden herself with unnecessary work coming from poor planning. In the space of her weekend reflection, an idea popped into her head that if she did some key reorganization at work, more progress would result, requiring far less of her time. In addition, she found that spending time in reflection and relaxation on the weekends felt so good that when she went to work on Mondays, she actually felt inspired at work and ready to pursue her goals.

A few months into her new routine, Maria couldn't believe how good she was feeling. At her six-month follow-up she was pleased to find that her vitals were well within normal range. In addition, she was delighted by the progress she was having at work and appreciated having more relaxation on the weekends. Both changes supported her overall desire to be a "grand innovator" in her industry, her fresh ideas inspiring both her and several of her colleagues. She also loved her Saturday mornings at home as they became her wellspring of rest and inspiration; these times became a weekend morning tradition cherished by her family.

Maria's experience – listening and responding to her body's signals of stress and physical need – is an example of *living into wellness*, and her wellness offered her plentiful energy to live into her inspired life. Maria's experience is a model of how to *live into inspiration* instead of making choices that lead to distraction (and The Bog) – in her case, illness and recuperation.

Allowing yourself enough mental and emotional quiet time – learning to pause and listen to your desires, your needs, and your longings in daily life – allows you to hear the voice of your own inspiration. Without stopping to allow your desires to emerge, or perhaps to hear the warning voice of your own discomfort, you become distracted and head down the path to *somewhere else*. On this path, you will surely end up in The Bog, distracted from the flow of native feelings and inspiration that are delivered to you moment by moment. Listen to the subtle cues letting you know you are veering off the course of your Grand Mystery – and take the time to realign with your spirit, the Grandest Mystery of all.

The Abundance of Inspiration

Many people struggle to find inspiration. They feel stuck in the crossfire of daily problems and begin to describe their lives in the language of scarcity, of fixing that which is broken, of urgency, and of fear. We sometimes get a lofty idea in an area where we would like to grow and expand, but then get sucked into the Zeigarnik vacuum, the obsessive pull on the human mind that calls us to spend our vital energy on finding things lacking or wrong, things broken and unsolved. With the pull of scarcity language and a focus on what's wrong, we get distracted from our inspiration. We lose sight of our purpose and once again bury ourselves in daily mundane and problematic details. How then do we maintain our inspiration and allow our ideas to creatively marinate and grow into our expanded selves?

There is no end to our ever-expanding inspiration. Day by day, if we ground ourselves in our Grand Mystery, reflect on the Quests with our anchors, and ask, "What's next?" then life will continue to roll out the red carpet ahead of us and invite us to join in the flow of life's river. Inspiration is an abundant resource with continual replenishment. It exists in every perception, in every thought, in every moment of every day. I encourage you to seek out and fully experience your native perceptions, thoughts, and feelings. Find your sparks – your unique inspiration – and allow your ideas to take root and grow. Commit to a life worth living and experience the joy of the never-failing *Process of Inspiration*:

1. *Esteem Yourself: Rest in the knowledge that "we are" (we exist), "we are a given," and "we get to pick" our future. No action needed.*

2. *Become Quiet: Empty and allow mindfulness to create emotional space. Empty the vessel.*

3. *Ask Important Questions: Explore "Who am I?" and "What comes next?" Then listen to the answers.*

4. *Marinate and Act: Allow your thoughts to root and grow. Always do what's next.*

5. *Look: For evidence of success.*

As you reflect and ask your way into your Frontier Adventure, you may have experienced the inevitable resistance that rears its unruly head: Doubt! It could be self-doubt, or the doubt of others, telling

194

you that you can't do the "it," that "what's next" of your inspired journey. The Golem may also, from time to time, grab at your ankles, but you now have the tools to use the *Language of Well-Being*, Debris Removers, and the gems of Native Experience to stay focused and move forward skillfully, without allowing distraction to derail your new adventure.

~

Thank goodness for your time on the "Bench of Reflection"! Recalling your Grand Mystery and noting that you are well along on your journey, you gracefully arise and reflect upon the anchors that drive you to inspiration. As your mind flits from family to career to wellness, hobbies, and everything in between, your heart warms as you appreciate each of your anchors. How lucky are you! A couple of your treasured priorities need immediate attention, but understanding the *Process of Inspiration*, you know the answers are only one question away!

In your feelings of joy, you begin to move slowly. First, you step right foot to the front, then bring forward your left (*I step into inspiration*); you raise your arms upward toward the sky (*I exist – in perfection with nature*). Next, you follow your bent elbow as you turn to the right, negotiating a full circle (*I become fully quiet; emptying my vessel*). This is pleasing! Next your arms stretch upward as if pleading to the heavens (*I ask an important question*); then you draw your hands down softly, laying them gently across your heart (*I listen to my answer*). Kneeling on the ground, tilting your head up toward the sky, you begin to sway and are enraptured (*marinating and asking, "What's next?"*). Holding the pose for several seconds, you are mesmerized by the apparent flow of your life and the delightful answers of what comes next.

Finally, standing back up with your arms outstretched from side to side, you first turn to the right, then the left, and then you survey everything around you (*Looking for evidence of success – there is plenty!*). Returning to a standstill, you bow a *Namaste* (*in gratitude for all that you are and for all that you will become*).

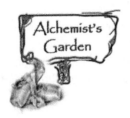 You have learned the steps, you are *Dancing with Inspiration!*

Alchemist's Practice

As a budding Alchemist of Experience, it is quite important that you learn how to allow inspiration to arise. The **Process of Inspiration** is a very straightforward approach for creating mental and emotional space that will allow your inspiration to arise. The biggest challenge is quieting your "monkey mind."

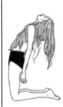

Process of Inspiration / or the Dance of Inspiration

1. Esteem Yourself
2. Become Quiet
3. Ask Important Questions – Then listen to your own answers
4. Marinate
5. Look for Evidence of Success

1. **Dance with Inspiration** – Bring yourself into a comfortably seated position on a chair, or on the floor. Closing your eyes, bring your breath into slow and easy inhales and exhales.

First...Esteem Yourself

+ Begin to mentally list those things you especially value about yourself. See if you can visualize or mentally hear yourself, as you connect with those things you value in yourself.

+ Continue to breathe with slow and easy inhales and exhales, continuing your thoughts of appreciation, for three minutes.

Next...Become Quiet

+ On your first exhale, imagine that you are breathing your thoughts out of your mouth.

+ As you inhale, imagine that you are breathing in fresh, clean spaciousness.

+ Repeat these exhales and inhales, with the same imagery, for three to five minutes.

Next...Ask and Listen

+ *Ask* yourself, "Who am I?"

+ Pause mentally and *listen* for your internal voice to answer.

(Note: don't force an answer to your question, simply *listen* to the words that emerge.)

+ Repeat the Question and Listen for the Answer for three to five minutes. You may come up with a different answer to your question each time you ask; this is quite natural.

Next...Marinate

+ Pick one of your answers from the above "Ask and Listen" – the one you like the best!

+ Imagine yourself in that role in *great detail*. What are you wearing? What are you feeling? What are your desires? Who is near you? What are you saying?

+ Marinate and deepen your visualization, your feelings, and your thoughts for three to five minutes.

(Note: The longer you "marinate," the greater your momentum in the *"right direction."*)

Next...Look for Evidence of Success

- ✦ Conclude your meditation by breathing comfortably for several seconds, or until you feel ready to open your eyes.

- ✦ Resume your daily activities as you normally would, but look for those things about yourself that you imagined during your meditation.

1. Make notes about your meditative experience. What did you like? What worked for you? What would you do to better tailor the experience for yourself?

   (Note: It often takes practice to become comfortable with this meditative practice and to learn how to listen for your voice within. Keep practicing...your answers will come because you are asking the question.)

2. Go through the meditation again, asking other questions you would like to explore about yourself. Here are some ideas. Just keep your questions short and simple!

   - ✦ What do I love the most?
   - ✦ How would I like this room to look?
   - ✦ How can I be loving to _____?

∞

Chapter 8

~

The Alchemist's Garden

"The purpose of life is a life of purpose."

–Robert Byrne

~

*"The mystery of human existence lies not in just
staying alive, but in finding something to live for."*

–Fyodor Dostoyevsky, The Brothers Karamazov

Learning the *Dance of Inspiration* from the young woman at
the entrance to *Alchemist's Garden* has been a very soothing
experience, rich with feeling and suggestion. Each step brings with
it new sensations arising from the depths of your body – within your
spirit – as you flow and reach in rhythm with a deep inner yearning.

"What do I dance to?" you wonder, "Don't I need some melody to
move with?"

Pausing your practice to ask the dancer what music she is dancing
to, you notice she has completely disappeared! In her place are
five small posts embedded upright in the soil. You are certain they
weren't there before, but on the other hand you hadn't asked the

question about dancing either. Tied neatly to each post is a small sack of seeds with a label that reads, *"Plant me when you know what I am."*

~

The perspective through which we view our world is a tricky business. Do we experience our lives from the outside in, or from the inside out? This distinction can be a crucial determinant of our inspiration and can greatly affect our long-term well-being. Living life from the outside in holds the promise that those around us will be pleased with us...whether or not *we* are pleased. We construct our lives on the desires of others – our parents, partners, bosses, or friends; we serve at the pleasure of those whose approval we need.

How many times have you heard a story similar to the man, let's call him Mac, whose father wanted him to become a corporate executive. So he became one. This would not have been his chosen profession, but he was making his father happy and he was very good at it. He woke up each morning with a dull ache of anxiety, spewing doubt and debris along his morning routine. He started each day with three hundred emails to slog through, and corporate politics (not the products' mission) drove his strategy to succeed. He drove his employees, as well, to do his father's bidding. His father held great pride in his accomplishments.

During Mac's doozey of a mid-life crisis, he decided instead to pursue his own passion. With a modicum of guilt and anger over his lost years in corporate slavery, he quit his job as an executive to become a symphonic harpsicord musician (his private passion!). When the announcement was made public, the entire executive team applauded him – applauded his strength of character and congratulated his ability to pursue his authentic interests. On the day he left the company, many others, driven in their careers like Mac, eyed him with envy.

Living from the inside out presents a very different perspective on how we can live out our lives. The source of our inspiration becomes deeply personal. Instead of being motivated to please others, in spite of our own desires, we seek to follow those interests and passions that are native within us. What happens, though, if we struggle to find those things within us that inspire?

In this chapter, *The Alchemist's Garden*, we will learn how to look within ourselves and identify our deepest sources of inspiration. Our sources of inspiration lie at the very heart of our Grand Mystery; they form the inspirational garden of life that quickens our hearts and that greets us with quiet joy each morning when we rise.

Seedlings

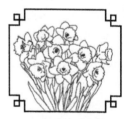

Looking around the Alchemist's Garden, on both sides of the curving path, you see all sizes and shapes of individual parcels, each seeming to tell its own story. Some plots are round, others are kidney-shaped; some have only seedlings, while others are overgrown and sprawling. Many contain both small seedlings and larger plants.

Alongside the plants in each garden are small posts like those now in your possession. Most of them have names, like "Shayna" or "Michael" or "Judith." Others have labels, like "house," or "music," or "poems." There seems to be no rhyme or reason.

Where do you begin to unravel this mystery?

We all have seedlings of inspiration in our hearts and in our minds. Although we tend to think of our lives as having a single Grand Mystery, in truth we have many. Like pallets of seedlings, we tend many areas of our lives out of love and a desire that those we cherish will grow and evolve into their own rich maturity.

My first palpable experience of a *seedling of inspiration* was when my son was "birth-minus-four-months." Several months into my pregnancy I decided to go crib shopping for the nursery. I was cruising the aisles of overpriced chairs and cribs and stopped at a crib that looked just about right. Then, like an emerging seedling of neonatal energy in my heart, I felt a new awareness, apart from me, that seemed like my son's conscious presence coming into existence. I imagined a small seedling arise from my heart and settle in my mind. There was no thought per se, only the physical and mental sensation of a presence to which I responded silently, "I promise I will take care of you on this earth." A small "seedling" of inspiration was planted in my body, in my own consciousness, and he needed tending and care.

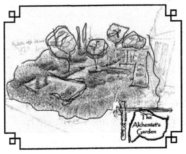

Since then, I have noticed many "seedlings" emerge and disperse in my life. They occupy psychic or emotional space in my mind; they often well up in my heart. Some seedlings are of people, others are of passionate interests. Some emerge anew, like my Granddaughter, that are small seedlings, while my son's initial seedling is now growing into maturity. My career is a relatively mature plant, now fully grown from its seedling of passionate interest that I have tended and developed with care for twoscore years. My husband is a relatively new sapling of inspiration: we are three years married, and this is still a relatively young growth. My wellness is a mature oak which brings me much strength, joy, and vitality. Piano playing is a scraggly vine, I don't spend much time tending it; I consider it outside of my garden, though I appreciate it when I can.

Each of these areas in my life has sprung to life in my Garden and requires tending to thrive. I love them all, and each brings me a wellspring of joy and inspiration that anchors me in love and safety as I journey. Other seedlings have come and gone in my garden – college, some old but not forgotten friends – and I expect there will be more changes as life progresses. But for now, I have a lush garden, my "*Alchemist's Garden*," that provides me a rich palette of colorful life from which I create.

These seedlings and more mature treasures, each providing a wellspring of inspiration, anchor us in our lives. They form a dense core of richness in our lives out of which our inspiration grows.

I am eager to share this idea with the Dancer — she is nowhere to be seen!

Preparing the Garden

What do the seedlings in our lives have to do with inspiration? The quick, accurate, and easy answer is *everything*! Our seedlings anchor us and help keep us focused on those things that are most important. It is easy to imagine what each seedling might look like in the life that we so deeply yearn for. Our seedlings form the foundation of desire and encourage us to create our own special roadmap (without distractions) toward the life we love. Recall that the process of inspiration requires to us to ask two very important questions in the space of quietude: 1) "Who am I?" and 2) "What comes next?" What would happen if, following the process of inspiration, we asked these two questions about each of our maturing seedlings?

First, we become quiet and acknowledge that we are the creators of our own lives. We take a few moments and empty our vessel; we embrace our innate sense of goodness and experience of self. Then, we choose one of our life's seedlings (or maturing growth) and ask ourselves, 1) "Who am I?" [in the context of that specific anchor] and 2) "What comes next?" We listen deep inside for an answer, a quiet knowing. As we marinate in the answer we imagine how the answer might look (if it were visual), or feel, or sound like. We could imagine the future reality and relish every moment as it approaches. Sure, there may be a couple of distractions along the way, but we examine them to glean out more of what we desire. Finally, we begin to look for evidence that we have begun our journey.

Here are some tips for planting the seedlings in your Alchemist's Garden. Notice how simple and effortless it is to create your garden, and how powerful the questions are in allowing your inspiration to arise. First, identify the five most important seedlings, or saplings – those people or things – that you care about the most. Focus only on five, more than that exceeds what we can easily manage in our busy lives.

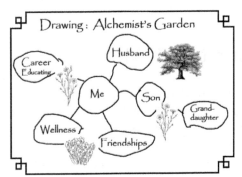

Drawing: Alchemist's Garden

Next, create a "bubble map" drawing that includes a circle for you at the center, and another for each of your seedlings or saplings around you. My drawing looks like this (OK – I couldn't leave out my granddaughter!):

Your drawing may look very different. Your seedlings of inspiration may be in different locations, or be of different sizes or shapes, they may have colors. Don't feel constrained about how to represent your seedlings, your favored approach will emerge through trial and error. Remember – trust *YOU,* make it yours.

After creating your drawing, select one of your seedlings to get creative with and begin to access your own inspiration using the *process of inspiration* and focusing deeply on the two questions above. As an example of the complete process, I will start with my "Son" sapling.

The "Son" Anchor – Following the Process of Inspiration

1. *Esteem Yourself*: I rest in the knowledge that I am perfect as I am today and I get to pick the future I have with my son. No prior history has been laid in stone and I get to pick how I would like our relationship to grow. No action needed.

2. *Become Quiet:* I go into my backyard, sit in a peaceful place and release my habitual thinking. I do this by sitting quietly, focusing on the sound of my own breath, and listening to the sounds in the yard. I allow my mental machinery, my thoughts, to be released as they arise. I allow a mindful state creating emotional space. I have "emptied the vessel."

3. *Ask Important Questions and listen to my own answers:*

   ✦ *Question:* "Who am I?" [in the relationship with my son] What is my Quest?

      Answer: "I am a loving mother and a life coach. My Quest is to teach him how to be the creator of his own inspired life."

   ✦ *Question:* "What comes next?"

      Answer: "I will create special "outings" with him a few times a month, and give him the space and permission to share about his life, his hopes and his dreams. As coach, I will offer support, and if it seems right, discuss options."

4. *Marinate and Act:* I will continue to mull this idea over in my mind and begin to visualize where and when we will get together, what will be enjoyable for both of us (I don't want to press conversation!) and allow him the permission and support to be himself. Doing what's next, I will set up hiking outings with him, meals together, and other get-togethers as often as time permits.

5. *Look for evidence of success:* After talking to my son and sharing the desire to spend time hiking with him, my son jumped on the possibility and would love to take hikes with me (success!). We scheduled our first hike.

6. *Repeating the process...Now I ask, "Then what's next?"* — "How do I ensure that I give him the space to share about his life candidly?"...And that internal dialogue, using the question of "What's next?" continues; I answer and mull the answers over in my mind to create the best possible scenarios.

What happens when we have a perfectly inspired idea, but we don't get the result we were hoping for? This happens to all of us as we learn and grow. Generally, the seedlings we choose are spot on, as are our Quests. However, the devil is in the details, as it is impossible to know in advance – or to control – events in our lives; we can only control ourselves! We don't know what we don't know.

Practice...practice...practice! Learn through trial and error, and each time you encounter a distraction, clear the debris using any of the Alchemist's Tools. Sustained attention to distraction will send you on a miserable journey to *Someplace Else.*

A friend's daughter, Liz, recently began her freshman year at college. She was excited and full of anticipation about the upcoming year, and appreciative that she got the classes and dorm that she wanted. All her "What's next?" quests about school seemed to be producing the results she wanted. In the "bubble map" drawing of her seedling anchors, one of her circles contained the anchor "Roommates" with the quest being to form a close-knit friendship among the two other girls she was rooming with.

Unfortunately, the two roommates that were assigned through the dorm admissions office didn't work out well for Liz. One roommate was a follower, which may have been okay if she followed Liz, and the other turned out to be quite a bully. Unfortunately, the "roommate that follows" followed the bully, Liz being left out of conversations unless she became a ruthless gossip. This was a big disappointment, and Liz didn't know where to turn next.

Knowing she needed to adjust her strategy, Liz revisited her original inspiration drawing, and felt the seedling "Roommates" was still desirable. She also reaffirmed her Quest to seek college roommates that could form close relationships with one another. At the question "What's next?" Liz sat quietly in the cafeteria, did her best to come into personal silence, and then used the "Debris Wiper" to wipe away any remaining mental chatter from her mind. As she envisioned the path before her she created a visualization about what she wanted in her mind's eye – she saw herself walking down the tree studded path on campus putting up a flier looking for "BFF Potential Roommates" to contact her. Liz talked to a number of girls and found two she thought would make great friends. They all met together and seemed to fit compatibly, at least for this freshman year.

Liz did four very important things as she continued her original Quest. First, she did not become distracted by her early less-than-perfect results to find friendships *and* roommates. Second, she confirmed that the "Roommate" seedling was still among her top five anchors keeping her Grand Mystery on track. Third, she re-evaluated her Quest to find roommates that could form close friendships to each other. She then paused to ask again, "What's next?" knowing she needed to make her Quest visible so others could respond. Finally, she didn't waste her time on meaningless options and mind chatter; she cut a direct path forward with a focused Quest for her flier: "BFF Potential Roommates."

Inspiration that is tied to your Grand Mystery *and* to each of your seedling anchors is a recipe for wellbeing and joy. Once you learn to clear the debris along your journey using the Alchemist's tools, the path before you is wide open for you to design, create, and build the life that you yearn for. Once you learn to keep your path clear and quickly remove useless distractions you will find there is much to learn and appreciate along the way.

Finding the Music

You have come so far! You have learned how to have a wealth of well-being as you journey to your Grand Mystery. You have embarked upon many quests in the Quagmire and have chosen the path less traveled – the Path of Inspiration. You have wrestled with stories, myths, and golems and you have cleared all the debris along your way. Looking behind you at your journey so far a familiar sense of accomplishment fills your heart. You have learned the *Dance of Inspiration*!

Finding the Alchemist's garden is a treasure in itself. It is filled with love, passion, and the people that give meaning to your journey. For the first time you feel anchored and supported in your travels, surrounded by all that you love. Perhaps there are a few scraggly vines here and there that need trimming or replacement, but now that you think about it, you know what's next. Your inner knowing tells you what's next and creates its own inspiration! Inspiration is surely abundant – it is everywhere you look, just on the opposite end of each distraction. Come to think of it, your distractions are beginning to recede quietly into the background of your life as the music calls you louder, and then still louder to dance with inspiration.

~

Lovingly you begin to map out your Alchemist's Garden. Recalling your Grand Mystery, and noting that you are well along on your journey, you begin to draw circles on the ground – this is the drawing of your cherished life's seedlings of inspiration. As you stand in the center circle of your drawing, the "ME" circle, your heart warms as you appreciate each of your seedlings and grounding they provide. How lucky are you! A couple of them need immediate attention, but understanding the *Process of Inspiration* you know the answers are only one question away!

Kneeling to the ground and reaching into your Knapsack for a pen you begin to label each post. With loving-kindness and compassion, you plant each seedling; already inspiration arises in your heart and mind for each one! Each seedling is a life affirming resource, inspiration at its best. Your *Dance of Inspiration* is well on its way!

Again, you dance! First, you step right foot to the front, then bring forward your left (*I step into inspiration*); you raise your arms upward toward the sky (*I exist – in perfection with nature*). Next, you follow your bent elbow as you turn to the right negotiating a full circle (*I become fully quiet; emptying my vessel*)...

Giggles pierce the quiet! Fragrant laughter penetrates your heart. Looking up, on the other side of the *Alchemist's Garden* is the Dancer ensconced in a joyous giggling huddle with – who? – her young family?

"These must be *her* seedlings!" you muse. Do you interrupt their huddle to inquire which music she dances to?

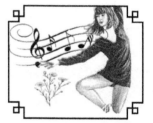

No need, you think, *I have found my own music* with which I will dance.

Alchemist's Practice

We draw our inspiration from those things in our lives that we value the most – our "**seedlings**." Masterful Alchemists select no more than five areas in life where they will dedicate their time. Any more than five dilutes your energy and attention.

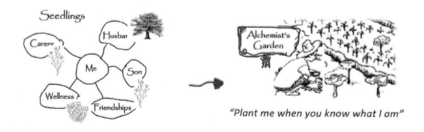

"Plant me when you know what I am"

1. Create a diagram for the 5 things you value the most in your life – your seedlings.

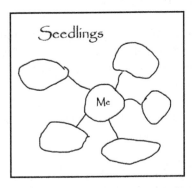

2. Pick one of your "seedlings" and use the Process of Inspiration to get clarity on how you are inspired to tend your seedling. Use the example in this chapter as a model.

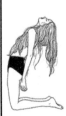

Process of Inspiration / or the Dance of Inspiration

1. Esteem Yourself
2. Become Quiet
3. Ask Important Questions – Then listen to your own answers
4. Marinate
5. Look for Evidence of Success

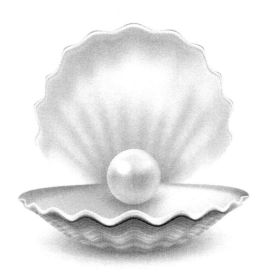

∞

Chapter 9

∿

Learning the Dance

*No problem can be solved from the same level
of consciousness that created it.*

–Albert Einstein

*The key to growth is the introduction of
higher dimensions of consciousness into
our awareness.*

–Lao Tzu

Standing back and admiring your seedlings in the Alchemist's
Garden, you celebrate with your personal Dance of Inspiration. You
have planted each seedling with commitment and care, and you now
wonder what all the negativity was about as you began your journey.
It is difficult to feel that your life is lacking when you sit in the middle
of your Garden among all that you have planted and love.

Inspiration – ideas – for each seedling flood your mind, including
potential quests and the anchors you have established en route to
your Grand Mystery. Yes, you are aware that there are a couple of
relationships that need attention, and you also have many ideas
concerning your career and home life for the future. For now, though,

you feel well-grounded in your life. You know it is your job – and your pleasure – to tend your garden.

It's hard to tell, exactly, how long you have been engrossed thinking about your desires and inspiration. Perhaps you're getting a little bored admiring your Garden, and you might realize that inspiration and ideas alone won't give you the life that you are yearning for. "Now what?" you ask; and in that instant, you find yourself back in The Bog coupled with your doubt, analysis paralysis and fear.

Living *from* inspiration sets us up to have a brilliant adventure, and this new experience can cause you to feel yourself teetering on the edge of a new frontier. As you begin to recognize these moments of inspiration, and marinate in their substance, you soon learn that inspiration alone is not enough to bring our dreams into reality. In fact, as we begin to identify, nurture, and nourish our inspiration, we quickly begin to encounter bottlenecks, or resistance, to furthering our inspired journeys. Perhaps you have self-doubt, or worry that your ideas may be rejected by family, friends, or coworkers. This is the time to use the Alchemist's tools to clear your path and protect your inspiration. Now is the time to rely on your own wisdom and understanding about yourself, others, and your environment. It is the time to prepare for what lies ahead: the positive and negative reactions from other people, the less-than-hoped-for results, and the challenges to your own self esteem.

Living an inspired life is not simple. It is for those whose resilience continues to be refreshed through communion with source, the core beliefs about yourself, and a strong understanding of how inspiration is turned into reality.

To navigate the gap between inspiration and creation, you must understand where you are in the *Process of Creation*. There are four distinct phases we go through to bring an idea into reality. The more we understand the purpose of each phase, and the activities we do in each, the more confidence and ease you will experience as you live into your inspired life.

The *Process of Creation* includes the activities we engage in and the state of mind, or type of conscious awareness, that is required at each phase. For example, if you have ever prepared to take a driver's test you might tell a friend, "I have to *psych* myself up for this!" What we mean by this is that we have to study for the test until we have a feeling of confidence that we will pass it. If we were to describe our state of consciousness we might say we are "persevering" through the test preparation.

Ideas evolve, and aspirations change. As they do this, it is reassuring to know where you are on the path to manifesting your inspiration and how you might mentally and emotionally prepare and execute each phase. The *Process of Creation*, of turning inspiration into reality, is exhilarating. Sometimes the journey may be arduous and filled with potholes, setbacks, and frustrations which can derail the best of Alchemists. However, with an understanding of how the *Process of Creation* works, it can radically transform your experience and your outcomes. Life becomes full of mystery, anticipation, confidence, and surprise.

Learning how the *Process of Creation* works in daily life is our exploration in this chapter. Inspiration is *necessary, but not sufficient,* for living into the life you yearn for. You must also learn how to take an inspired idea from conception to manifestation and bring it to life within the bounds of your life, our society, and the prevailing culture. Finally, you must learn how to manage the many undesirable outcomes and the resistance from the status quo we will encounter as we give birth to a new reality. Chapter 9 is intended to introduce you to that process of creation.

~

Sitting in your Garden, surrounded by those things in your life that give you an abundance of joy and inspiration, you once again look around all the parcels in the Alchemist's Garden. Some are neatly tended; the weeds have been cleared and the old growth removed. Others look like they need tending, trimming, and clean-up. Some may need additional nourishment from their owners as their leaves wither with neglect. Many look utterly abandoned – perhaps the owners are captives of their own Golems!

Looking upward and around the Alchemist's Garden you notice – *were they here before?* – a series of Terraces rising up from the base of the garden and extending up to the very top of the hillside. They are all trimmed and pristine, each terrace holding a unique character quite different than the others. Each Terrace is a seeming *world* unto itself. Each of these Terraces represents one of the phases in the *Process of Creation*, and your next step is to explore them.

Looking for the Dancer, you find her waving to you from the highest Terrace. But by now you are not so surprised!

Welcome to the Terraces

Living into inspiration requires us to understand and master *how* we create our own reality. We always create reality from our own inspiration; but as we adventure out to create our desired reality from inspiration, we must know how to navigate the different levels of consciousness – our own internal states of mind – that we will experience. These are the Four Worlds contained in the four Terraces. Similar to any landscape, you can picture the Terraces as having four unique worlds (or levels of consciousness) that you might ascend, with the highest Terrace being the furthest from your reach as you begin.

Perhaps you can remember a time in your life when you had a great idea and felt the joyful and engaging feelings that accompany this inspiration. Then you brought your idea forward to family members or colleagues who didn't share your level of excitement, or who perhaps even tried to shut your idea down or sought to change it to fit their own desires. Notice how your feelings quickly shifted from inspired excitement to disappointment or discouragement. What happened? Where did your excitement go? It was as though you had just entered a new world of gloom and doom; your mood abruptly fell, as if the curtain had been lowered on what should have been your best performance.

Then, remember another time where you may have had an inspiration, perhaps a do-it-yourself type of project where you just sank your teeth into the "doing" of the project. You've got a design in your mind (or maybe on paper), you gathered the needed materials from around your house or from the store, and you charged ahead, engrossed in your project. You were focused on creating and delivering a completed project born from your initial idea. Somehow you have moved from the world of inspiration, your idea state, into the active world of doing. You have moved from the world of thought into physical reality. *Doing* is a mental state quite different from *imagining*. Proceeding to the *doing* of an inspired idea involves a complete change of consciousness. You are ascending to the next higher world on the Terrace.

Your level of consciousness often changes without your giving it any thought – you are living in the moment. This may be described as a change in your feeling state, but moving from imagination to actively gardening is much more than simply a change of feeling or body movement. Your *level of consciousness* must change in order for you to move from one world to the next on the Terrace.

There are four distinct levels of consciousness on the Terraces which carry an inspired idea forward from inception to completion. Generally, when we conceive of an idea, we are in a state of imagination where our rules about reality are suspended and new possibilities are free to arise. This is the World of Creative Reality, its own world of thought and emotion. Next, we might debate internally with ourselves whether the idea is a good one or not. The conscious activity in this World of Discernment has a very different quality than it does in the World of Creative Reality. Proceeding further along our creative path, we start to build out the idea into the physical world, perhaps by telling others about the project to get advice, by picking up some "how-to" books if we need them, or by doing research on the work of others. This is the World of Mastery. On this level of the Terrace, we gain direct and needed skills, construct detailed plans and models, engage with others, and experience successes and failures. Finally, as we give birth to our completed project, you are able to produce and experience the fruits of your labors. This is the World of the Manifest, where we experience the outcomes of our initially inspired idea and share our results with others.

Each of these four levels of consciousness (which the Alchemist envisions as Terraces arising out of the Garden) has its own specialized purpose in the process of creation. Understanding each of these Worlds will help you understand and navigate a clear route from one state of consciousness to the

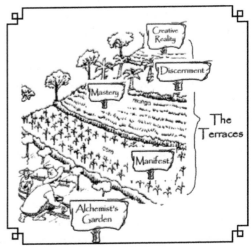

next, from an inspired idea all the way to a manifested reality. This knowledge provides guidance for the experiences you may encounter and will help you think through how best to proceed. Although the states of creation generally work in a sequential flow, top to bottom, there is a very dynamic interaction between all of the stages. The interactions between the states of consciousness form the *dance of creation* itself.

The World of Creative Reality

Looking upward to the Dancer on the uppermost Terrace above the Alchemist's Garden, you imagine the air must be most rarefied and pure. It is so close to the sky and the heavens you think, "The dancer must be dreaming up something divinely inspired, maybe even fanciful...!" You can still hear giggles from where you are below – how did the dancer get all the way up there?

The root of inspiration is the information that our senses perceive and translate from Source energy; we combine new and old information to form fresh ideas – our inspirations. Inspirations have their native physical, mental, and emotional components; they are new vibrational experiences. In the *World of Creative Reality*, your consciousness is one of free-roaming thoughts and ideas. In creative consciousness, you can imagine anything and there are no real or imagined boundaries about "what's in" or "what's out." The experience is one of a waking dream, with unhurried possibilities and ideas crossing our boundary-free mindscapes. There is no judgment, no best/worst scenarios, just a timeless state of imagination where possibility abounds. You may be sitting in meditation, staring at a blank sheet of paper, jogging, or doing routine tasks where our minds are free to wander. It is a state of relaxation and calm – a place of internal enchantment that will spark new ideas.

Not long ago I was shopping for an anniversary present for my husband. As I was browsing a book and arts store looking for ideas, I noticed a striking painting of the tree of life, each quadrant of the tree painted distinctively with a lovely poetic phrase for each of the four seasons: spring, summer, fall, and winter. Immersing myself in the concept of the picture, I could feel the little electrical charge of inspiration: a shot of "approach-me" adrenaline. I felt excited, and knew my husband would love this painting. It was a physical, mental, and emotional reaction that was additionally buoyed by other creative arts surrounding the picture. Following the inspired reaction, I felt happy and excited about the prospect of giving it to him on our anniversary. I cultivated the inspiration, imagined giving it to him, and felt the delight – in that moment – of lovingly presenting it to him.

Inspiration is the *starting point* of living into inspiration, the *beginning* of creation. As we translate perception into inspiration and idea, we are drawing upon source energy for stimulation and mixing it in with our own life experience. Native inspiration often feels enlivening as you sift through ideas, imagining their ultimate *reality* and picturing their eventual manifestation. If you dive into the inspiration you can experience the feeling – somewhere in the manifested future – of how you will feel when it is completed. We think about what inspires us and begin to apply our own wisdom and understanding to the idea. We can imagine native inspiration as being an inviting lump of wet clay; we dip our hands in the silt and begin to give shape to our ideas. We think about it, mentally enact possible outcomes, and access our inner experience and wisdom ("Ah, this is good!"). We mull things over and shape our inspiration into an even more robust idea. This is your inner knowing, the basic stuff that is the basis of our thought reality – the blueprint of a future in the physical world that we wish to create.

It wasn't long ago that I was taking a yoga class and heard my instructor tell me, "You would make a great instructor." I was in the yoga studio, among friends and other aspiring yogis, when the inspiration to become an instructor sprang to life. I felt a surge of excitement, took in the studio's calm environment, and could feel the internal "vibe" of being a yoga instructor. That vibe, or vibration, of being a yoga instructor had a sense of competence, physical mastery, love for the learning process of students, and a fair portion of eternal grace. I felt pride and a sense of future and purpose. I could imagine myself spending time in a studio, teaching; I could imagine myself at the venerable age of ninety-two, teaching students to hold a "Crow Pose" and a "Jump Back" – and I could see and hear myself offering commentary on the Yoga Sutras and other philosophies. It felt good. *I felt inspired.*

This is the time to seize the inspiration as your own destiny and focus your attention on it; let it marinate. Neuroscientific research on memory tells us that it takes from ten to fifteen seconds for information retained in short-term memory to transition into long-term memory. In addition, the more ways we capture the inspiration (by picturing it, feeling it, etc.), the more synapses are formed. Therefore, it is important to seize the idea (visualize it, feel it, hear it, draw it, etc.) for at least fifteen seconds in order to allow it to transition into long-term memory. The longer you focus your attention and thoughts on the idea, the more robust your memory of it will be – along with your vision of your inspired future. With *less* than fifteen seconds of thoughtful attention, however, your inspiration will only remain in your short-term memory, where it will atrophy into a fleeting memory as it retreats.

As my inspiration to become a yoga instructor was born, the visual, mental, and emotional reality deeply resonated within me – the vibration of who I was to become held an intoxicating thrill. Game on!

With the inner knowledge of the path before me, I knew success was a given. The future was mine to shape, to form into my reality, to create a new direction for myself and the others in my life. Persistent imaginal destiny in the absence of conditioned debris will transform your life; once you think it, it is done.

These moments of inspiration are to be valued, cherished, and nourished. This is "the Stuff" of your inspired life. Feel the vibe of the future you, see the future *you* in action, play out your destiny from all sides, and know that through your own inspired intention, the universe will yield to you exactly that for which you are asking.

This unfettered, creative, excited, and inspired state of consciousness is like none other. There are no boundaries, no "shoulds," no "you cant's." There is simply the thrill of creative inspiration and an imagined future. It is fresh, and it feels good. You have now begun your inspirational journey, standing at the apex of the Terrace known to the Alchemist as *World of Creative Reality*.

Once again you think of the Dancer high above, bringing an imagined tomorrow into reality.

The World of Discernment

From the World of Creative Reality, we move to a state of consciousness where you give deeper thought and consideration to your inspiration. This is the World of Discernment, where you consider your inspired intention, including its pros and cons, and discern whether the ideas that flow from it are in concert with your Grand Mystery. You consider if the inspiration is in keeping with the deepest intentions for your cherished seedlings, your treasured contributions, and your core beliefs. It is here that you entertain a more thoughtful exploration of what your inspiration entails and seek to ensure that it is in alignment with your inspired future, your contribution to the world outside of you. No matter how small or large your contribution to the world will be, the impact on yourself and others is important in determining how to proceed.

In the World of Discernment you debate, asking, "Will creating this reality make me joyful? Will it benefit others, or harm them? Does it matter? How does it fit into the world around me?" You are full of thought, defining the boundaries of "what's in" and "what's out." You test the goodness of the ideas against your *feelings* about them. Using the Alchemists Measure, we ensure that we are going in the *right direction* – toward our treasure! – and we ask, "What's next?"

As I sorted and sifted through my thoughts and feelings about becoming a yoga instructor, I began to feel a growing sense of commitment, not only to my own physical and spiritual development, but also to the enrichment of my students. This became very important to me and directed my education into deeper aspects of spiritual development as a complement to the physical practice. The more I sifted, the more I imagined, the more I spoke to others about my idea, the more inspired I became. From the central theme of my life's mission – to create wellness through spirituality – I knew this direction would bring goodness to me, students, studio owners, and my family. As for my husband, he began to hold pride in my accomplishments and spiritual development. For my son, I became a positive role model for connection to self, inspiration, vitality, and wellness as an aging parent. I know, too, that this will ultimately influence his own thoughts about vitality in life and aging.

There is no "right size" for a contribution. I have a friend who is inspired to make her bed extremely well every day; sheets tight, blanket smooth, and pillows carefully positioned to create a sense of artistic flair. She rests assured she will feel a sense of beauty and comfort when she crawls into bed at night. As she prepares to sleep, she will enjoy a well-made bed in a home she loves and sleep with an extra bit of appreciation and calm. She will likely be a nicer person to those around her in the morning. This is a profound goodness in simplicity.

Sometimes an inspiration is colossal, like Diana Nyad's desire to swim from Havana, Cuba to the Florida Keys. Not only did she realize a lifetime dream of swimming the 110-mile channel at the age of sixty-four, she became an international role model for becoming "all you can be" and helped to open new cultural relations between the US and Cuba. Her deep desires from childhood and the actions she took later in life became an inspiration for others on a grand scale, through the message she delivered: "Live large."

It's not the size of the inspiration that counts, it's the results. The gratification of a goal accomplished or an inspiration realized delivers a fulfilling sense of esteem, knowing you are the driver behind your own choices and your own life.

Time spent on the Terrace in the World of Discernment strengthens your sense of internal conviction, enhances your inspiration with depth of meaning, and calls you to powerful acts of defining – and wrestling with – your desired contributions.

Suddenly you hear a thunderous clapping from above! Looking up, you see the dancer, giggling with others nearby. They are giving each other a round of high fives! Surely, they have reached consensus about something.

The World of Mastery

Watching the Dancer's experience, an uneasy stirring begins to percolate in your heart, a yearning with a bit of hesitation for what you imagine in your inspired life but have not yet realized. In your mind's eye, you can now visualize the growth in your seedlings, inspired projects getting underway, and the expansion within you. As your yearning unfolds further and your inspiration evolves into real possibility, you begin to look and listen for a sign urging you forward...perhaps the birds will sing a melody of praise, or the breeze will whisper, "Congratulations."

Above, wafting down from the upper Terrace, what you hear instead is a cacophony of argument piercing the quiet of your imagination! Looking up to your dancer, somehow now on the second Terrace, you hear her arguing with the other travelers. "I thought the dancer was well on the way to her personal 'Splendid Days,' but apparently she is not," you think. "This is *not* good!" Since you are a budding Alchemist, you must learn what has happened.

Having experienced the exhilaration of inspiration in the World of Creative Reality, and after validating the goodness of your inspiration in the World of Discernment, the World of Mastery awaits you. Consciousness is much different in this world. It is at this level of the Terrace where the physical, emotional, social, and mental work gets done in order to bring your inspiration to life. In the World of Mastery, you gain the real-time skills and experience needed to achieve your dreams; you learn to master relationships with those around you, and you spend your time working toward manifesting your inspired life.

Of course, there is *a lot* to learn in this phase of creation. Sometimes your expectations and desires are a bit hazy or unclear to begin with, and initially they may produce less-than-satisfactory results. Perhaps those people around you see the flaws in your efforts, disagree with your direction, or channel other negative thoughts and energy your way. These are challenging events and can transport you directly into The Bog – if, that is, you are not alert.

In the World of Mastery your consciousness is that of a *learner.* The World of Mastery requires you to learn the skills necessary to construct your desired outcomes. These include not only specific, hands-on skillsets, but also general leadership skills, such as the ability to: influence others, manage change, learn communication skills, and successfully create productive relationships. Much of your life is conducted in the World of Mastery. You experience successes, failures, and travel steep learning curves in this World, while emotions take us on a rollercoaster of ups and downs.

Even in the World of Mastery you continuously ask, "What's next?" You feel, think, do, and learn – in that order. In the consciousness of

Mastery, you focus on real-time progress and problem solving. You will need perseverance and receptiveness to new ways of thinking, doing, and being. But you also need to stay wedded to your deepest self and do your best to remember and apply lessons that come to you along the journey.

Great skill is needed in all areas of your life; however, *the first and foremost priority is mastery at remaining in alignment to your true self.* Staying centered in your *Core Beliefs* and following your inspiration towards your Grand Mystery will keep you afloat, inspired, and optimistic.

This is a critical phase in realizing your inspired life. *You must remain in close alignment with your deepest, most substantial inspired self. Your internal compass is the most important asset you have in getting through this part of the journey successfully.*

Whenever you fall out of alignment with your connection to source and inspiration, you will feel pain. You will suffer from the crevasse that is formed between your authentic self – native experience and inspiration – and your pursuit of distraction. It's like saying, "I want to lose weight," and then binging on a big meal and dessert. The gap between your inspired desire and your subsequent action creates a painful internal contradiction!

Self-imposed suffering that arises out of this crevasse between your aligned self and the attention you pay to distraction can be fatal to living an inspired life – if it is not recognized. But once you recognize the experience, you can "feel" your way back into alignment, your centered self filled once again with inspiration and esteem. Return to your Alchemist's Garden, apply the Alchemist's Tools, and ask each seedling anew, "Who am I?" and "What's next?" That's it. Returning to your inspired life is always one question away, if you'll pepper your efforts with a bit of courage.

Once I had left the corporate world in order to pursue my inspired mission of bringing wellness through spirituality to others, many of my closest friends that supportively began my journey with me became ardent critics. I had dreams of creating a physical space that would be "the most perfect place to spend an afternoon," where we could teach people how to live into their inspiration through joy, fun times, and community. I also dreamt of publishing a guide to help people align themselves to their deepest selves and live into their inspiration. Yet my dearest friends kept bringing their own fears of failure into the conversations. They weren't shy about telling me all the things they thought I was doing wrong, their worries about my strategies, and the use of my time. They weren't quiet about my choice of business partners, and they disguised their own fears as "constructive feedback."

These are the most challenging of times when, through peer pressure, fear, or mistakes we reverse ourselves on the path going in the *right direction* and begin to go *someplace else*. But remember, it is *we* who *make the choice to be distracted,* it is *we* who *choose to step away from living into our inspiration,* and it is *we* who *choose to live our lives in reverse gear.*

Anne, a dear friend of mine, had spent many years struggling with her weight and pursuing a private practice in early childhood education. She was deeply inspired to help language-impaired children and desired to experience and appreciate her own sense of sensuality and beauty. She was a loving and sensitive soul who spent her lifetime giving support to others, but through her upbringing had learned to meet other people's needs before her own. Although this was an endearing trait, it had not worked in her favor. Anne had strong career aspirations and was intensely creative, but when other people discouraged her, or wanted her to change to make them happier (yes, it happens all the time), she would give in and become a people-pleaser. She would abandon her own inspired life in the service of keeping the peace, or mollifying those who needed her to be something other than who she was. She would shut down and ignore her own inspired thoughts; for her, the thought of not meeting the needs of other people seemed selfish. She was deeply concerned that her friends, and especially her husband, would stop loving her.

Constricting or shutting down our own natural inspiration is difficult, and it actually takes energy to keep our inspired thoughts from rising to the surface. That is why when you are feeling constricted, you also feel tired or fatigued. It is similar to the experience of holding your hand over the gushing end of a hose; tremendous pressure builds up behind your hand in the walls of the hose, and it takes persistent effort to continue to hold the water back. However, after years of habit restraining your native instincts and feelings, this repression begins to feel natural. In Anne's case, as she held her inspirational energy at bay she became irritable and began stress-eating to keep her inspiration – and her anxiety – tamped down. Clearly it was not a decision born of desire, but rather was a choice made from a place of fear and insecurity. Anne complained often about her high stress levels and overeating, but at the time, she believed she needed to suppress her creative energy to maintain her relationships.

It is easy to see how acting out of fear, or any other negative-conditioned feelings, can deplete your energy and your ability to live into inspiration. In fact, it marches you in a negative direction away from inspired living and further entrenches unhealthy habits.

Once Anne was exposed to living into inspiration and had a "mental model" of Native Experience, contribution, and continuous alignment with her deepest self, her life began to expand in many directions. She slowly became able to sustain her inspiration and to renew her self-alignment (her seedlings and "what's next"). She learned how to return to the World of Creative Reality to center and reestablish her inspiration, and she became able to hold on to and marinate into her inspired life for longer periods of time. She learned to restabilize into her Core Beliefs and Grand Mystery quickly when her inspiration and creativity were challenged, and she has gone on to develop an innovative approach to the treatment of children with learning disabilities.

As Anne began to achieve a stronger sense of alignment with source, and her inspired self, she started to allow her inspiration to emerge in other areas, such as diet and nutrition. She learned to more readily identify moments of inspiration, marinate in them, parse out their depth of meaning to herself and others, and deliver them to the World of Mastery for execution.

Inspiration *always* feels good...and the more you have, the more you want. It is profoundly engaging and energizing to experience your truest self. In fact, the feeling of alignment allows your constrained energies to be released into the natural flow of your life. Tight muscles release into meaningful and directed action, feelings and thoughts begin to flow forward effortlessly, and endorphins release into the brain causing a natural high – or *joy*.

As Anne gained Mastery in her new direction, she began to watch cooking shows and learned that cooking could be an art form. She planted a new "seedling" in her *Alchemist's Garden* of making her food artful and well balanced, and she began to vary the themes and plating design of her kitchen creations. Her stronger – and more frequent – relationship to her true self put her in touch with what she described as "streams of inspiration" in other areas of her life. She began to feel positive forward movement in other areas of her *Garden*, watching each of her "seedlings" grow. It was as if a "Go" sign had been ignited in her heart, so much so that at times she needed to slow down in order to not overcommit herself; instead, she would allow herself the necessary time to catch up with – and grow into – this new, bigger version of herself. Much to Anne's surprise, her family and many of her friends also grew, inspired by her changes – further rooting Anne in her new life adventures.

From time to time, we may lose connection with our own alignment to source. These are times when our inspired thinking is interrupted, and we get knocked off center. We are all so well trained to live out of alignment that it doesn't take much for a grumpy spouse, a rebellious child, or a controlling boss to refresh all of our previously conditioned thought and behavior patterns. Losing alignment to source occurs more often when you are initially beginning to live an inspired life. You might come in contact with discouraging people, frustrating events, and – of course – old habits, but this is where you can exercise your new skills and build up *inspirational muscle*.

Practice the art of realignment every day; the World of Mastery is full of opportunities.

"Ah," you think, "the Dancer is learning how to solve a problem with other sojourners! That's what that arguing – debate, really – was all about." You now understand they are learning in the World of Mastery: mastering how to work *together.* They have made it this far, and you can sense their commitment as their voices quiet and they get to work. Gazing up one last time, you see them in a group hug!

The World of the Manifest

As you desire so shall you receive! Through the Worlds of Creative Reality, Discernment, and Mastery, your inspirations will come to life. There are also many things to learn on the bottom Terrace, the World of the Manifest. As you enter this world you start to notice the things you have manifested. They may appear as you had expected, or they may show up in some very unexpected ways.

Consciousness in the World of the Manifest is grounded in our everyday experience of physical reality. You are on firm ground: you know what you see, feel, and touch. It is rich with enjoyment and can be peppered with disappointment. From your realized life, your grounded consciousness, you can decide what to change and what to leave alone.

As you gaze up at the Dancer, you see an unusually artistic-shaped picnic table on the lowest Terrace. Its surface is olive wood in a kidney-shaped form. The legs of the table arch upward from the ground until they meet together, halfway between the ground and the table's surface; then they fan out again in curved, branch-like configurations until they reach and support the tabletop. The dancer, along with the other travelers, are laughing and celebrating the formation of their final product. It is indeed innovative, and quite stunning.

Suddenly the dancer pauses in surprise when trying to sit at the table. There are no chairs! The design was wonderful and the table turned out beautifully – but no chairs were designed to sit in!

You guessed what the dancer was thinking. "What's next?" And at that instant the dancer disappeared from the Terrace. Looking high and low for the dancer, you see her re-emerge on the top Terrace – which you now know as the World of Creative Reality. The chairs are in their inspirational phase.

Not too long ago, I was inspired to create a life of public speaking about wellness. In the World of Discernment, I knew this would contribute to improving the lives of others. It felt good (great actually!) to act in accordance with my deepest self, share my knowledge, and be who I was inside and out. At the time, I was teaching yoga and began to bring a deeper wellness philosophy into each class. I had entered the World of Mastery, and as I tried out new topics and approaches, I learned what worked and what didn't. My students offered me much learning in return. Their questions were sensitive, and their desire to learn was deep. Not too long afterwards, my husband bought me a book on yogic character traits which was a perfect fit for what I needed in order to add further depth to my classes. I read it daily and incorporated it into my work. My short yoga talks began to grow into longer talks, and before I knew it I had enough material to begin preparing full-length lectures. It was as if the Universe had conspired to help me put all the components of public speaking into place; new people came into my life, and new opportunities presented themselves often. At times, I had to put opportunity on hold; I needed to slow my progress down – too much was coming too fast.

When you engage in the feelings and consciousness of your inspired life and live into your expanding self, you selectively attend to those things which you intend and desire. Perhaps it is the manifested equivalent to quantum physics – like attracts like. My inspiration and energy for becoming a public speaker on wellness brought me students who were interested. They brought me more knowledge, which in turn gave me more to speak about. I sought out more teachers and they became part of my life, books arrived at my door, and my inspired evolution was well on its way in the World of the

Manifest. The experience was surprising and absolutely a Frontier Adventure for me!

Sometimes, however, you might manifest things you didn't know you wanted. There are those things in our lives that might make you ask yourself, "How did I manifest ___?" However, if you are honest with yourself and look at what you created, you can usually trace the outcome back to its native desire.

I had spent many years as a senior manager on a very technical program in the aerospace industry. Although I loved the job, it was extremely demanding and difficult. I was working ten-hour days and many weekends, yet in spite of it all I loved the experience. During that time, I was also going through a divorce and found the transition very difficult. My days were intensely busy, and my evenings and weekends were lonely. I was learning how to be a single parent. Then, as though the fairy of difficult times dropped a package at my doorstep, my company went through a reorganization and I was transitioned to a position well below my capabilities.

I hated the job. My successful career took a nose dive. I was bored and unchallenged, and I felt like I did not belong in this lower-skilled position. It was a blow to my ego. One discouraging day I took a minute to pause and ask myself "How did I get into this position? What did I do to bring this on?" A deeper, wiser, and knowing self answered: "I am tired. I need time to recover [from the divorce]." In that moment, I connected to the wisdom of source and spirit and understood the wisdom behind my manifestation. A physical release of energy and resistance washed over me and I felt myself, for the first time in months, moving in the deeply aligned direction of my own life's current. I felt *relief*. My perspective shifted, as my "boring job" became an *opportunity* for a much-needed respite.

There are times in life when I pause, reflect, and notice what I have currently manifested. I look in the rear-view mirror and ask how I got to where I am. In *theory,* you *know* you create your own life, but like me, your real-time connection to the Native Experience that got you there is hidden beneath your myths of "shoulds" and "can'ts." This is the time to pause, empty the vessel, and ask your knowing self, "Who am I? What am I feeling? What inspires me right now?" Stop, become quiet, and listen to the answer from source and spirit.

In the World of the Manifest we actually get what we asked for – *without fail*. We are either aware of asking, or not. When we are unaware of our asking, it feels like "things just happen to us," like we are swimming upstream against a forceful current. We may feel out of control, unlucky, unhappy, disappointed, or perhaps victimized by others. Our bodies may be telling us we are going *someplace else* through headaches, painful backs, or frequent colds. We feel the need to exert ourselves to get what we want. But when you are mindful of your Native Experience, your deep asking, and your aligned "knowing," you simply do what comes next and progress surefootedly through life. Sometimes, as in my example above, you might experience the need to rest, take a break, or maybe even pivot direction. Your distress is a clear indicator that you are not in alignment with your deeper self. Listening to your deeper wisdom is an imperative.

It feels exhilarating to allow your energy to flow without inhibition or resistance, to live into your inspiration, and to expand in your most cherished directions. At these times, when you trust in your Native Experience and take your next step forward, you are being all that you can be – as you step into the life you yearn for.

The Dance of Creation

Everything in life has its own pace and flow; that's what makes *living into inspiration* the adventure it is. As you move between the Terraces, through the Four Worlds of Creation, you experience a series of unique and different levels of consciousness. Each level of consciousness, each World of Creation, has its own purpose, its own vibrational or physical experience, and its own result. You might think of this as a dance through the Process of Creation as you: (1) give birth to inspiration; (2) discern its contribution to your lifelong journey; (3) master the skills and solve the problems necessary to build toward your desired outcome; and (4) bring it to life as you intended. Let's summarize the dance through the Four Worlds:

1. In the *World of Creative Reality*, you receive source information from the environment around you, and spirit – your deepest self – gives birth to new inspiration, calling you forward towards your Grand Mystery. When you are in the World of Creative Reality, your level of consciousness is infused with dreamy imagination; you may feel a sense of freedom or lightness, since here reality is suspended as you imagine unbounded "what-ifs." There is no right or wrong, no problem to solve, no people to convince – you are experiencing the joyful interpretation of source energy into an inspired idea. In the quiet of your wakeful dream, new realities are born.

2. In the *World of Discernment*, you assess the likelihood of bringing your inspiration to life and examine whether the inspiration has merit in achieving your inspired outcome. Here you measure, discern, and clarify your inspiration. You may decide it is of key value in achieving your desired contribution, or perhaps, as you mull it over, it may appear to be a distraction or a bit off-track. In the World of Discernment, your level of consciousness becomes evaluative, you measure pros and cons, and you ground your inspiration in probabilities. The dreaminess that arises in the World of Creative Reality is transformed into practicality of thought, balanced with the love and compassion that brought forth the initial inspiration. You may experience this level of consciousness as having both constrictive and compassionate qualities. It is the "go/no-go" level of thought and emotion, either moving the inspiration forward to the next Terrace of creation – or deciding to do something else.

3. In the *World of Mastery*, you learn the skills necessary to bring your inspiration to life. You live and learn, so to speak, as you begin to build toward your inspired outcomes. Perhaps you need skills of influence or leadership. Perhaps

you need to build interpersonal skills, take a course, or learn the skills of "doing." In the World of Mastery, you learn and build, experiencing successes and failures and learning from each. Your level of consciousness is that of problem-solving, progressing, and sometimes repairing your wounded ego – you celebrate the good times, or prepare yourself for the next effort. Your emotionality abounds in the World of Mastery as you conjure inspiration and give birth to its manifestation.

4. In the *World of the Manifest*, you see finished products, or perhaps your incremental byproducts. What you desired in the World of Creation is now your reality. Sometimes your creations are exactly what you had imagined, and sometimes they miss the mark. But you can be sure that each success or near-miss will result in a return into the World of Creative Reality. If you create the reality you had imagined, you will naturally return to your wellspring of inspiration for new ideas. If you miss the mark, you will return to the world of inspiration and ask, "What's next?" This then allows your deepest self to embark on the next leg of the journey. Consciousness in the World of the Manifest is observant; you register Native Experience about what you have manifested, and you are launched back into new inspiration.

    If you find yourself making excuses in the World of the Manifest, being self-critical or otherwise emotional, be aware that you have returned to the World of Mastery, where your conditioned emotions have re-emerged and must be addressed. As you master removing your debris, these will no longer hold you back from achieving in the World of the Manifest.

Imagine the Dance of Creation as performed by an architect hired to build your home. The architect will sit down with you and ask what you would like built and where you wish to build it. They will gather your unique needs and desires – your requirements – and retreat to their offices to imagine a design that fulfills your wishes. This is where you (the customer) and the building site together serve as a significant source for the architect's inspiration. The architect now asks, "What is the overall result, the central Quest of this home?" He entertains answers such as "the perfect home to raise a family," or maybe "the perfect home to entertain in." The architect now has at their fingertips your desires and needs, a sense of your personality and interests (gathered from their experience with you), an understanding of the property shape, size, location, and neighborhood – along with a more holistic sense of the intended outcome for the finished home.

The architect, taking all the source information from you and the environment, then asks the question to himself, "What does this Quest suggest creatively?" As the architect empties the vessel (clears his mind), inspiration and ideas spontaneously emerge in the World of Creative Reality. The architect, responding to your needs and the world before him, will imagine one or more design ideas, perhaps draw them out, and allow their consciousness free inspirational rein.

Having pictured these designs, the architect will then move into the *World of Discernment*, where the ideas will marinate and questions will be asked about the merits of each, mulling each one over for the goodness of the design and making changes, if needed. "Will the needs and desires of the client be met by these designs?" "What could be missing?" "Is there anything that wouldn't work?" "What are the unknowns?"

Still in the *World of Discernment*, the architect may invite you to a meeting where you will see the design options and evaluate potential designs (marinate and discern). At some point a determination will be made as to which design, if any, you and the architect will move forward with.

Once a decision has been made to move forward with a design, the architect will enter the *World of Mastery*, where his skills will be put into action by drawing a building plan, detailing the materials, costing out labor, and so on. You and the many people the architect works with will require strong interpersonal skills as challenges, negotiations, and other situations – good and difficult – emerge.

Working with builders, contractors, and regulatory agencies, your home will be erected. As it enters its completion phase and emerges into the *World of the Manifest*, the project will become complete – an inspiration brought forth into reality.

Of course, this is a straightforward example of the Process of Creation, but it is through clear illustration that we understand the basic form of how we live into inspiration and manifest the lives we yearn for.

Living into your inspiration always provides unexpected twists and turns. You may be inspired to be a good partner, a supportive parent, run a marathon, write a book, or become an executive; however, you will always bump up against some resistance or troublesome situation as you make your way to your dreams. You will experience false starts, setbacks, or partial results. This ebb and flow of progress is natural; expect it. It is the nature of creation, the way the river flows as it makes your journey exciting.

Every inspiration and idea plays out its own dance as it works its way from concept to creation. The *Four Worlds* on the Terraces are your playground, and it is both a challenge and a joy to navigate when you are equipped with a map of the territory and plenty of opportunity for practice.

In the next chapter, we will take a deeper look into each of the *Four Worlds* and what they feel like in our own bodies, minds, and spirit. We will also look at how we exist in relationship to our environment. Dancing within the Four Worlds is not a linear path to creating inspired lives. We weave in and out of each world; our state of consciousness shifts day to day, and this continual journey is truly a dance with inspiration, the world, and all that we are becoming. It truly is a dance where sometimes we trip over our own feet, but, at other times, we gracefully dance through to the finish line.

∾

Looking for the Dancer you see an astonishing sight. Six olive-wood chairs have been placed around the table – equally as unique! The beveled legs of each chair are curved to match the natural shape of their branches. A brilliant design.

In the blink of an eye, the dancer disappears – then, just as suddenly, she reappears on the uppermost level of the Terrace, returning again to the World of Creative Reality!

"Ah," you think, "she must have asked 'What's next?'"

Alchemist's Practice

There are four distinct **levels of consciousness** that bring an inspired idea from its inception to its completion. Each of these four levels of consciousness has its specialized purpose in the process of creation. The Alchemist of Experience becomes a master at understanding each level and understands that the **Process of Creation** flows from the **top terrace to the bottom**.

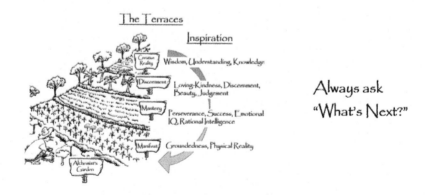

Always ask "What's Next?"

1. Think of a creative project that you have completed in the past. It could be a family project, an artistic piece, something related to

your work, or something involving a community activity. Describe the project briefly below.

_____

_____

_____

_____

2. Taking a look at your *creative process* for the above project, and see if you can describe each stage of its development.

Level of Consciousness: In the World of ...	Describe what you felt, thought, and did at each level.
Creative Reality	
Discernment	
Mastery	
Manifest	

∞

Chapter 10

~

The Dance of Four Worlds

*"If you want to find the secrets of
the universe, think in terms of energy,
frequency, and vibration."*

–Nikola Tesla

"The energy of the mind is the essence of life."

–Aristotle, The Philosophy of Aristotle

"How do I get to the top Terrace, the World of Creative Reality?" you ask yourself. After having seen the Dancer rematerialize from one Terrace to the next – *you didn't see her hiking* – you wonder how she managed the feat.

Sitting under an oak, having learned about the different levels of consciousness that accompany each step in the Process of Creation, you begin to study what happens in each of the Four Worlds. If you study diligently, perhaps you can get to the different Terrace levels. As they say, knowledge is power.

Sitting in the Alchemist's Garden, admiring your seedlings as you study, you conclude that this approach isn't working. You know the steps by heart – what's wrong?

Knowledge is helpful, but experience is a necessity when engaging with the Four Worlds of Creation. Perhaps you remember the first time you saw snow fall? For me, there were no words to describe the experience. My feelings and thoughts became expansive, and perception fanned out beyond my physical boundaries as my awareness extended out into the very snow itself. I was transfixed in a state of suspended wonder as the beauty of the white particles sifted down to earth. Looking up to the clotted grey-white clouds, I saw millions, maybe even billions, of snowflakes floating down like feathers surrendering to gravity. The white ground and snow-dusted trees completed the magical effect, forming the image of a storybook's winter cottage.

Notice how the experience gets lost in the phrase "It snowed this morning," or "You should have seen the snow – it was amazing." No words can adequately convey the depth of wonder or the experience of awe so rich it brings tears to your eyes. How can you adequately convey such an experience to another person? They must experience it themselves, firsthand. Anything less than having the direct experience comes up dishearteningly short.

The same can be said of the Four Worlds of Creation. Each world is rich with texture that words cannot adequately describe. Words can direct your attention, or your awareness, towards what to look for, but not until you see it, feel it, and walk in its energies will you fully comprehend the experience.

In this chapter we will explore our conscious awareness in each of the Four Worlds. Each world has distinctive characteristics, its own set of vibes, and an interplay of vital energies or feeling states. Dip your toes into the experience of each world; try on the energies and begin to understand the Terraces as you live it in real time. This chapter will help direct your attention toward each level of consciousness and invite you to delve into your own Frontier Adventure.

First, we will examine the idea of our *"energies"* – we will learn how they are more than any single feeling or thought. Next, we will explore our basic energies *beginning* in the World of the Manifest, then move upward to the World of the Mastery. Next, we will move upward again to the World of Discernment, and then finally arrive at the World of Creative Reality.

It is important for Alchemist-in-Training to understand that when we engage in *self-reflection* we learn about ourselves from bottom to top, from the World of the Manifest upwards to the World of Creative Reality. However, when we *live into inspiration,* we Dance with Creation from top to bottom; that is, we *start* from the World of Creative Reality and work downwards to the World of the Manifest.

As you read through the examples given along our journey through the Four Worlds of Creation, I invite you to write down your own real-life examples for each of the four worlds. There is no better way to learn about your different levels of consciousness than by

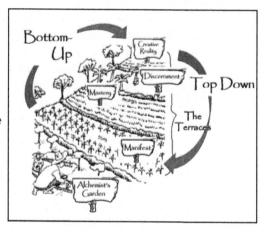

reflecting on your own life, *inside* your own body and mind, and taking time to explore your experience through writing or other artistic mediums.

Knowledge is no substitute for experience.

Understanding "Energies"

We all carry our internal *energies* around with us every day. Our *energies* can best be described as a mood, a general state of mind, or a "feeling tone" we may be experiencing. Some days we are aware of our energies, especially when an event triggers a stronger-than-usual reaction; other times we may be aware of low-grade moods that we can't really identify.

There are times the energies we experience are so strong they actually override our logic and biological functioning. I will use such an example as a teaching point to clearly illuminate the experience of an *energetic state.*

Years ago, my son was in a car accident shortly after his seventeenth birthday. He was found by his girlfriend about midnight, standing barefoot beside his totaled car on a remote country road; he did not know who he was. At the time, I was living four hours away when I received his girlfriend's late-night panicked call. As she described what was happening, I felt the blood drain from my head and my mind went completely blank. (I experienced it as feeling "white" inside.) I didn't have any prior experience that matched that feeling to use as a point of reference, but a jolt of hot fear shot through me as though I had just been hit by lightning. My mind started racing and I feverishly began asking questions: "Is he hurt?" "Can he talk?" "Can he walk?" "Does he know where he is?" You can imagine a parent's reaction!

I stood by as a local friend brought my son to the hospital. I couldn't sit still; my body ached with adrenaline. I paced the floor fearfully back and forth, with a racing mind and a pounding heart. My perception of time shifted into slow motion as I awaited word from the hospital. Ready to act – in an exceptionally high state of arousal – I was amped; mobilized in a state of "doing" in the World of Mastery.

Imagine the state of mind you would be in during a similar type of situation. There were five elements contributing to this highly aroused state of consciousness:

1. The *physical* Native Experience of arousal–emergency; elevated heart rate, tight chest, flight/fight response, native fear

2. The *meaning* I gave to the situation – deep concern for the safety of my son

3. *Conditioned emotion* – fear about car accidents and injury

4. The rapid *self-talk question: "What's Next?"* – and its answer: *"Wait!"*

5. An extended "wait" period – *time* – in a heightened state arousal

Taken together, these five internal encounters produced a state of heightened awareness that created an energy state of gritty *perseverance*; I had to *persevere* through this stressful period of time until I had enough information to act. I was in the World of Mastery – mobilized and ready to respond – as I awaited further information about my son. I had to remain strong to cope with a very difficult situation. Fortunately, my husband was present and provided a strong source of support for which I will be forever grateful.

It seemed like an eternity, until finally I got a call letting me know that my son had bruising, a concussion, and amnesia. It was expected the amnesia would diminish as the concussion subsided. I was able to speak to my son, who glibly told me, "If you want to know what happened, you're talking to the wrong guy!"

The situation, thank goodness, resolved favorably. I drove south to see my son early the following morning. His memory had begun to return, and his bruises were relatively minor. The powerful energies of the previous twenty-four hours began to subside, as a curtain of relief washed over me.

Although this is an extreme example, it is intended to serve as a bold illustration of an *energy* – in this case *perseverance* – a vital energy found in the World of Mastery. Perseverance is, as are other energies, a *combination* of internal and external events: *Native Experience, conditioned emotion, situational discernment, the environment, and experience over a period of time* come together to create an overall mood or general tone.

States of consciousness in each of the Four Worlds contain their own characteristic energies, or feeling tones, that are recognizable once we begin to learn the territory. Much like the Dancer, we can shift from one level of consciousness to another by asking simple questions and waiting for our own inner voice to answer.

Once we have awareness of our energies and the level of consciousness we are experiencing, we can train ourselves to navigate the Four Worlds of Creation with ease and mastery. Then we can proactively engage with our inspirations to live a richer and more meaningful life.

As we live into inspiration, that is exactly what we do. We come to experience and engage with our own energies, understanding they are each different from one another – each facilitates an important aspect of the evolution of an idea or intention from inspiration to creation. Each energy has its own unique and internal physical, feeling, emotional, mental, and spiritual characteristics. Each has its own role in realizing a dream or manifesting something desired. All energies are precious and valuable, no matter how they may appear at first glance.

We must experience our *energies* firsthand – how they feel and how they affect our bodies and minds – and then give thought to the role they play in our lives. Plato once said, "An unexamined life is not worth living." While this is a bit of an overstatement, it does point to the idea that there is more to life than what appears on the surface. As Alchemists, the more we learn about and engage with our energies, the richer our lives are.

The Dance of Four Worlds is an embodied experience as we become internally aware of our own bodies, perceptions, energies, and actions. Because this is a *self-reflective* exploration, we will begin in the World of the Manifest and dance our way up the World of Creative Reality. With a bit of experience, and some trial and error, we will be Dancing in the Four Worlds in short order.

Energies in the World of the Manifest

In a very concrete way, we see, feel, and touch things in the World of the Manifest. Our worlds are populated with shaded forests, vast oceans, beautiful shorelines, colorful flowers, and so much more. There are all sizes and colors of people, alongside thousands of species of animals and other critters. We enjoy cars, streets, shopping centers, movie theatres, and so on. We have our bodies, our fingers, our toes, noses, and arms. We have fast food, soda, alcohol, and chocolate. We have Facebook and YouTube. The World of the Manifest is a veritable marketplace of things to see, feel, taste, touch, and hear. Every manifestation is the result of someone's desire. The "stuff" of the physical world presents us with the *artifacts* of inspiration.

How do we embody and experience the World of the Manifest? Our five senses are our receptors: we see, touch, feel, smell, and hear the manifest; these senses inform our relationship with the manifest. Jasmine blossoms on the vine display exquisite, glossy leaves with small, white flowers. The texture is slightly rough, the blossoms smooth and slick. The vines have a sweet and pungent smell, yet we are not drawn to taste them.

We have two other perceptive channels that add to the richness of our five senses. A sixth sense, called "interoception," provides us the ability to feel our bodies from the inside – like our heartbeat, or a full stomach. Finally, "mirror neurons" in the brain provide us with a seventh sense, an *empathic response* to other people's feeling tones – such as when we find ourselves sitting in the same posture as a colleague, or how we can "feel" another person's sadness or pain. We perceive and respond to *all* of our real-time experiences no matter how small.

From our perceptual experience, the World of the Manifest elicits a feeling within us that may be positive, or perhaps may repel us. In the manifest world, there are no conditioned feelings, only the direct perceptual feeling/thought experience. A skunk's odor repels us. We don't have to stop and think about it; the feelings are direct and immediate. The sound of a harp may be sweet to our ears as the melody draws us in.

Thoughts also abound in the World of the Manifest, yet they are simple thoughts originating from Native Feelings: The mountains are beautiful, the fire is hot; someone's energy is negative or it is positive. In the World of the Manifest, thought is immediate, it is primal, it is natural, and it is unhindered by past experience, fear, regret, or anxiety.

The World of the Manifest provides us with vital experiences that can launch us into action. An alarm clock can bring us back into worldly consciousness from a deep sleep, the sound of a streetcar may inspire a rhythm, a good joke can trigger another, or the sound of an emergency siren can make us immediately pull our car over to the side of the road.

The "stuff" of the manifest motivates us into action. Perhaps we experience only a reflex, as when a doctor taps below our kneecap and our leg jerks reflexively. Or perhaps we quickly hop up into the world of Mastery where a conditioned thought or emotion becomes triggered. In the World of the Manifest we are inspired to draw near, or pull away from something in our environment. It is our base experience: no judgment, simply the world as we receive it in the here and now.

Psychologists and philosophers have urged us for centuries to live in the "now." The World of the Manifest is that world. There is perception, native feeling, and initial thought. Period. It is simple and elegant, positive or negative, our environment inviting us to come closer or move away. In the World of the Manifest there are no life struggles, only the world in its purest form.

We can become constricted in the World of the Manifest by shutting off the flow of perceptive experience. Strong thoughts or emotions can pinch off our native experience, causing a loss of sensitivity to (or awareness of) our immediate environment. Intense fear, anger, or even excitement can tamp down our native awareness as we attempt to protect ourselves from intense experience, or as we become preoccupied with other thoughts. We become unavailable to the "here and now" and miss the richness or our environment – we are *someplace else.*

When I heard that my son was in an accident, I shut down experiencing events in the present as I focused one-pointedly on his safety. When we constrict in reaction to an event in our present experience, we are usually resilient and return to our unencumbered selves in a short period of time.

However, sometimes we constrict the flow of experience in a habitual way, forming patterns that are not healthy or adaptive. Imagine the husband who is bothered by the chatter of his wife. Perhaps he becomes steeped in TV, becoming oblivious to his wife's communications. How many times have you heard someone say, "He just never listens to me," or, "She doesn't really *see* me." Shutting down our "here-and-now" awareness can become a pattern that has a sizable impact on our lives.

Persistent constriction is a red flag for wellness as well as for living into inspiration. If we selectively ignore our awareness in the World of the Manifest, unfelt perceptions can eventually fester into stomach aches, vascular constriction, and other physical or mental ailments. Over time, constricting our perceptive awareness can become a lifetime habit with a high price to health and well-being.

Relationship problems, physical symptoms, and other constrictions are our body's signal that a very fundamental constriction in the World of Manifestation is at play. Stop, listen, and learn about your "here and now."

~

Perched under the Oak, you begin to reflect on the nature of your consciousness in the here and now. You notice that you are easily preoccupied with the Dancer and how she seems to appear and reappear on different levels of the Terraces. A bit of angst grips your chest because no matter how much you study the Terraces' "levels," you still aren't moving.

Focused on your worries and problems, you arrive at a stunning conclusion, "I may be sitting in the World of the Manifest – under the Oak – but my consciousness has just moved into the World of Mastery."

In that moment of self-reflection, you return to noticing the ground you are sitting on, its firm support, the rich, red soil and the strength of the tree's base and snaking roots. Looking upward you see the leaves slowly flutter in the breeze. The air smells fresh, and you notice how vitally alive you suddenly feel. In the World of the Manifest, life is good!

Just as quickly as you returned to awareness in the World of the Manifest, your worries and angst once again intrude on your "here-and-now" feelings. With your new awareness of shifting consciousness, you can tell you have slipped into a different state, into the World of Mastery, surrounded by your conditioned thinking.

Energies in the World of Mastery

Our energies reach a stronger vibration and our emotions rumble in the World of Mastery. We move from the physical and immediate perceptual world into the realm of the non-physical. We experience our conditioned emotions and thoughts; we experience the joys of victory and the agony of defeat. In the World of Mastery, we are rich with emotional texture, vibrant communication, love and relationship, passion and desires, work and perseverance. We live our day-to-day lives in the emotional and skill-based "doing" World of Mastery. It is the conditional world of "what is."

We all have a multitude of feelings about the jobs that we have, our family, friends, and acquaintances, and the quality of our relationships. We endeavor to learn new skills and fine-tune the ones that we already have. In the World of Mastery, we are the engineers of the world around us. As we continue to learn and grow into being more capable and competent people, testing out new skills in daily life, we often find success...and at other times get results that we don't want. The World of Mastery is brimming with challenge, with feelings of success or failure that uncover our strengths and challenges. We are offered untold opportunities to improve, to "up our game."

Challenge greets us daily. When I was working in the corporate world I would go in each morning and create a "To-Do List" for the day. I would take a blank piece of paper and draw four quadrants on it. In the first quadrant of the page, I would list the tasks I needed to complete during the day; in a second quadrant, I would list things I needed to complete within the week; in the third quadrant, I would list relationships I needed to nurture; and I would leave the fourth quadrant blank for notes.

Starting with my tasks for the day, I could read each one and feel the pangs of anticipation: "Write sections 4 and 5 of a procedure" – *Dread*, it's hard to get started; "Get buy-in on presentation" – *Excitement,* I love meeting with my sponsors; "Meeting with Boss" – *Anxiety,* too much political tension.

When I reviewed my goals for the week, I would do the same. I would remember where I left off on each goal and look at the challenges that needed to be resolved by the end of the week. Whether I was aware of it or not, I was setting up an emotional mindset for the week to come driven by past experience and future anticipation.

When I got to relationships – the hardest quadrant for me – I would stop to think about each relationship. Some relationships were a pleasure and brought me delight. Some relationships were political, and I would struggle with how best to handle them. The politics at work were never easy. I would make notes in the fourth quadrant to help me think through my challenges.

We all do some sort of planning every day or so; as we do this, we can see how our emotions arise as we review what we will be doing. How many of our negative and positive emotions come from our stored memories, our conditioned responses? Probably eighty percent or more. There is no better way to get a glimpse into your conditioned feelings than listing down and responding to the things you are doing in daily life. We get a glimpse of the lives we are living; many of our conditioned reactions spontaneously rise to the surface.

Imagine coming home after a long, hectic day. What list of tomorrow's to-do's are you reviewing in your head to make sure you don't forget? What feelings of anticipation are you experiencing during your review? If you are negatively anticipating something at home, like a cranky spouse, do you find yourself preparing a "cranky defense" before you arrive? Were your expectations accurate?

The World of Mastery is filled with landmines, challenges, and hoops to jump through. But once you begin to master the skills needed in this non-physical world, you begin to feel capable, competent, victorious, grounded, and satisfied.

The artifacts of The World of Mastery are your emotions, most of which are conditioned responses layered atop our native feelings in the "here and now," which is the World of the Manifest. In other words, the emotions are the recycled experience of past events where thought has intervened and added a second layer on top of our Native Feeling.

I remember when I was in my early twenties just learning about the complexities of romantic relationships and dating. I had gone out on a couple of dates with an intelligent, entertaining, and handsome man in whom I was developing quite an interest. On our third date, he very sweetly let me know that he had no interest in me.

I remember the feeling as though it were just yesterday. I could feel my heart sink, then I felt a deep appreciation for his honesty and willingness to be upfront with me. These were instantaneous feelings, my *native thoughts and feelings* as the conversation spontaneously emerged and just as quickly faded. The experience happened in the World of Manifestation – experience, perception, native feeling, and thought.

That evening, however, my thoughts and feelings in the World of Mastery began to kick in as I started to process the event. I began to feel rejected and started to look for what flaws may have turned off this lovely man. I was too fat, my clothes weren't chic, my personality probably flat. I started to feel inadequate and unaccepting of myself. Then I began to get angry with my date, diagnosing that he was probably afraid of intimacy or didn't have much experience dating.

I'm fairly certain we have all been in similar situations. In my pursuit of a lasting relationship, something had gone wrong. I deeply appreciated this gentleman's honesty and the actual experience was quite painless; However, upon reflection I had noticed many emotional and mental barriers that I replayed from previously learned mental models of ideal men, openness to intimacy, standards of dating dress, etc.

The World of Mastery is a vast territory, and it's where we spend a majority of our time. It contains thousands of lessons about how to master the challenges of the world and emerge confident, resourceful, and successful. Life in the World of Mastery requires honesty of feeling and thought, diligence in examining the resistance that confronts our deepest desires, and perseverance in never giving up on our heartfelt dreams.

Each time we navigate through our own resistance and learn the lesson being taught, we give birth to a better version of ourselves. Perhaps we learn the skills of surrender and intimacy, allowing for deeper relationships. Perhaps we try on new skills and, when successful, create new things – perhaps a completed design at work, a piece of art, or a beautiful memory with our children.

In the World of Mastery, we become capable and competent adults. Our depth of emotion matures; our hard-earned skills enable us to produce astonishing products in the World of the Manifest, and we begin to enjoy the fruits of our perseverance and effort.

~

Reflecting under the oak about "doing" in the World of Mastery is a good learning experience! You now know that your worries and concerns revolve around gaining stronger skills of Mastery, in this particular case your worries center around learning about your various states of consciousness and energies. You decide to practice using the *Debris Wiper* to move habitual thought patterns out of your way...so you can learn how to reliably descend into the sweet World of the Manifest – your calm reflective spot under that shady oak in the Alchemist's Garden. You want to be able to control your states of consciousness and also allow them free rein. You want *both* skills; practicing is a must!

Experimenting with turning your *Debris Wiper* on and off, you begin to gain control over moving from conditioned thinking to Native Experience. Next, you practice mastering the *Alchemist's Language*, so you can move yourself to more positive states of emotion and thinking. Next, you allow yourself to settle comfortably into the World of the Manifest where practice and perseverance has given you satisfaction and confidence. Your Native Feelings are far less frightening than your conditioned emotions.

Pausing in the World of Mastery, you congratulate yourself in mastering these two states of consciousness. From Mastery to Manifest!

"Ah," you think, "knowing when I am shifting awareness is good?"

Energies in the World of Discernment

In the days following my unsuccessful attempt at a relationship and my efforts to become a better person, I began to experience a soft, compassionate feeling that was heart-felt for my personal struggles.

It felt like a deepening of my lesson in relationship, an immersion in compassion and self-care.

That same week, as I walked to the bus stop on my way to work – still feeling the raw sting of disappointment and the grief of rejection – I sat down on a bench beside an unkempt man. Perhaps he was homeless, a conclusion I came to from the clothes he was wearing and his lack of self-grooming. A bow wave of compassion swept over me as I imagined that this man's beautiful soul must have been ruefully damaged in some way, and that he had not yet found his way back to self-respect. The day was richly overcast and heavy, which, in an unspeakable way, lent itself to the soft, low vibration of sadness and compassion. It was a moment in time that marked a developmental milestone in my own life – the experience of feeling a profound, compassionate caring for another.

The World of Discernment moves us to a higher level of caring and compassion that results from deepening experience in the World of Mastery and gradual emotional maturation. It is a world filled with loving-kindness for ourselves and for others. It invites us to reflect on a world that is bigger than ourselves, a world that has deep implications for the betterment of our lives...and for humanity; it invites us to examine what might be in the best interests of ourselves and others, in a grander scheme of conditions beyond just "me."

In this area of our lives, we *balance* issues that we hold dear for ourselves, our families, and our communities. There is a healthy tension between what is right or wrong, enough or not enough. This is the world in which we develop what the Buddhists call "right thinking." We have two or more conflicting alternatives that we need to choose from, and here we weigh and measure the goodness of our potential actions.

I used to see a man at the entrance to my grocery store with a sign saying, "I am hungry, please spare some change." Naturally, my initial instinct was to give a dollar to help a hungry guy – even though his belly looked like he ate quite a bit. I could always feel the little devil and the angel each perched on one of my shoulders arguing amongst themselves: "The man needs food," then, "The man is a cheat." What is the process we go through to resolve the dilemma? We assess our perception of his actual need versus our cynicism. Perhaps we question our cultural ethics to donate to the needy compared to our own financial status.

The problem was easily resolved one day when I overheard two grocery store employees talking about the beggar. Apparently, one checker saw the man enter the store early morning dressed quite well. He went into the restroom and emerged a few minutes later in tattered clothes and messy hair. My moral debate was resolved.

However, there are no right or wrong answers. We make the best decisions we can based on the facts at hand and the experience we have gained in our lifetimes. In the World of Discernment, we learn the boundaries of our personal values.

We have all had relationships we may have questioned for ourselves. We weigh the goodness of a decision to get into, or out of, a relationship. I had a bumpy relationship many years ago with a genuinely kind man who I had very deep feelings for, but he had very different parenting values than me. Much to my friend's chagrin, I didn't tightly control my son's intake of green vegetables; I was not a parent prone to criticism. Although my friend did not cross any significant parenting lines, our values did not mesh. When my small family was together I could feel the mismatch in the tone of some of our conversations. Also, in watching my son's body language, I knew that years spent in such a relationship would be harmful to him, ultimately harmful to me, and in the end harmful to all of us.

It took me months to weigh the issues and to discern what would be in the best interests of all us individually and as a family unit. It was simply a wrong action for me, in the long run, to continue the relationship even though it met many of my immediate needs for relationship and connection. Once the decision was made, it was as though a heavy weight had been lifted from my heart. In the wake of the decision, a sense of beauty and compassion for the three of us took root in my soul, and the flow of my life's river felt (thankfully) restored. After much thought and discernment, the path forward that was in alignment with my own desires and values had been forged.

We weigh, we measure, we balance, we discern; and in balance we bask in the beauty of our choices. In the World of Discernment, we wrestle with our alternatives, define our values, and strengthen our path from compassion to spirituality.

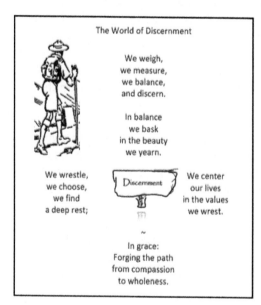

The World of Discernment

We weigh,
we measure,
we balance,
and discern.

In balance
we bask
in the beauty
we yearn.

We wrestle,
we choose,
we find
a deep rest;

Discernment

We center
our lives
in the values
we wrest.

~

In grace:
Forging the path
from compassion
to wholeness.

Whatever the issues, whether they are personal, interpersonal, community based, or global, the World of Discernment directs our decision-making and determines what paths our lives take. With attention focused on "right thinking," we learn to master compassion, loving-kindness, and thoughtful discernment to make the best lives possible for ourselves and for those around us. The artifacts of the World of Discernment are our deep-seated values and the boundaries of right thinking.

There is a breathtaking result that appears when we balance judgment and compassionate choices: the tender recognition of native beauty, even in a world of difficult choice. As we sift through the never-ending business of resolving dilemmas and making sound judgment, we are transported to a deeper awareness of the magnificent complexity of our world; when successful, we get a sense that we have done a "goodness" in the world, no matter how big or how small. We get a gentle view of a bigger picture, a world bigger than ourselves.

~

Contemplating the Dance of Creation in the shade of the oak, you begin to realize the powerful nature of your energies. Although you have experienced them throughout your life, you can now see the different states of consciousness you've always had but paid little attention to. It's as though you would float from one state of consciousness to another, from one World to another, with no distinctions about what you were doing. You have been operating on automatic pilot – no wonder you have felt the world was creating you rather than *you* creating your own world. You now realize you have always had the power to create the life you yearn for, but weren't aware of how to access it.

Noticing how unsettling it has been to not understand your own internal currents, you now realize that learning the skills of the Alchemist is illuminating the path before you in a very new way. You are beginning to feel more control and confidence in shaping your future and uncovering your Grand Mystery.

Pausing in this moment of reflection and epiphany, you drink in the elegance of the universe and revel in its magnificence. Learning the Alchemist's skills, you begin to feel a multi-terraced balance and beauty in your life.

"Ah, this, too, is good?" you think. Then whoosh! ...the feeling of beauty transports you upward, into a different and timeless state of mind – the World of Creative Reality.

Energies in the World of Creative Reality

In the World of Creative Reality, we experience our lives through the deep vibration of spiritual feeling, a powerful inner knowing based on the continually maturing *understanding* of our lives and the *wisdom* that we have gained from experience. You may have caught a glimpse of this world when you notice your gut feelings about something – an intuitive inner knowing. In the World of Creative Reality, our consciousness rises far above our practical day-to-day lives, and we see the world through the *timelessness* of source, through the eyes of our own perceptual awareness, and through the wisdom of our lessons learned. We become witness to, and connect with, the Flow – the longer game of our own life. We become aware of the current of our inner river, the deeper nature of our journey, with expanded insight into where we are headed...towards our deepest desires.

This is the world that mystics seek to embrace; it is a natural state of consciousness that has its connection in source energy, and that we all have the ability to access. Many of us have short glimpses of this world during moments of peak experience or heightened sensitivity. It is the birthplace of our own spiritual awakening; that deep inner space of knowing born of wisdom and understanding.

We gradually grow into the World of Creative Reality, testing our gut feelings and developing a keen reliance on our connection to source and to our intuition. How many of us have reflected on a past experience to see if an intuition was correct, or notice that we made a bad decision because we didn't listen to our gut feelings? We test, we learn, and we grow into our spirituality.

Remember that we received early training from our parents, teachers, and others, telling us to listen to authority instead of to our own feelings and intuition. The intuitive capabilities and spontaneity that we once had – and now see in very young children – are great reminders of the "powers" we now need to recover as adults. Our enculturation is valuable and important, but as we reach into maturity we must not allow it to sentence us in the prison of our adulthood.

We often live unaware of our imprisonment. Perhaps you recognize some of these familiar phrases we often hear that provide an indication that we have been jailed – that are cut off from our intuitive selves:

+ "Just be yourself" (as if you shouldn't – or couldn't!)
+ "I'm not creative"
+ "I'm not spiritual"
+ "Silence makes me uncomfortable"
+ "I can't be selfish"

Many years ago, I was on a consulting gig for an engineering firm in Southern California. Our mission was to work with management and employees in the hope of discouraging unionization. As part of this process, we spent weeks interviewing employees to better understand their discontent and to present a plan to management for improving employee relations. For a while things went along smoothly, but after about a month of work I began to feel an uneasy feeling deep in my gut that something wasn't right, that communications with employees were changing almost imperceptibly; I couldn't put my finger on it, but something wasn't right. I thought about bringing up the topic with the CEO, but I thought I was feeling a bit oversensitive; other consultants weren't having the same experience. I discounted my feelings and proceeded on as planned with the team, but the feelings continued at a low, steady level. A few weeks later my firm was pulled off the job. Apparently, the company's employees had indeed interrupted the flow of communication ultimately sabotaging the consulting effort. They successfully strategized to maintain their progress toward unionization.

As I looked back on what had happened, my gut instincts were firing early warning signals that I chose not to trust. I was relatively young in my career and didn't understand the value and accuracy of my deep perceptions. Had I known how to act on such instinctive information – had I possessed a stronger wisdom and understanding for acting on my gut instincts – the situation might have been averted.

The World of Creative Reality allows us to ingest subtle vibration from source energy. It is experienced as a deep-seated knowing and is the result of clear understanding and earned wisdom. If we had been taught to trust our deepest instinct and intuition early in life, our lives would likely be very different than they are today.

How many times have you heard that voice deep within, felt an intuitive knowing, and not done anything about it? Our Creative Reality is within us, always. Our deepest selves have the immediate knowing of our life's flow; we are at constant play with the divine source energy and perception we all possess, but only slowly do we learn to trust and consistently gain access to the deeper parts of ourselves. We must stop, look, and listen to the flow of our own lives. We must be sensitive to source energy and release ourselves from our bondage to "clock-time" in order to access the powerful inspiration that we all possess.

There is an orderly progression of emotional and mental development starting from the World of the Manifest and extending through each World of consciousness...until we are ready to harness our full experience – and our full potential – in the World of Creative Reality.

We enter the World of Creative Reality gradually, and often quite randomly, as we gain mastery in the preceding areas of our lives. As we enter higher levels of consciousness, we might experience unusual moments of clarity; we might have a creative experience that feels inspired (with a poem, a piece of music, or other art) and that seems to *create through us* instead of being the usual result of laborious effort applied to a challenging task.

When I had first moved to the Bay Area, I was experiencing a great many of these events. I recall waking up one morning, dozing in and out of sleep, truly enjoying that liminal space between sleep and wakefulness. In that quasi-conscious sleeping/waking state, feelings and events I had been mulling over seemed to get mixed with an energy that brought poetic words in blocks of thought to my thinking. I grabbed a pen and paper at my bedside, and with my eyes closed, lying in my sleeping position, I documented the words that literally came through my mind and directly onto the paper. The result was a deeply sensitive poem that seemed to write me – I simply documented what came through.

The experience was exquisite, gentle, and sweet, filled with words and feelings of knowing that were far removed from my normal daily routine. Thus began a new period when many poems "wrote me" and other inspired experiences occurred that let me know there were other realities to which we have access.

I do not believe this is a "mystical" world available to only a rarified few, but a consciousness that everyone has access to when they are ready. It is in the consciousness of Creative Reality where our level of wisdom, understanding, and knowing taps into the larger world of source energy, where we can experience the divine. Once there, we can become attuned to mastering that consciousness as profoundly as we can experience the worlds of the Manifest, Mastery, and Discernment. Even greater than mastery, it is *where we become able to create our own lives out of clear and present inspiration.*

~

In the quiet afternoon shade of the old oak, you realize you are daydreaming in the World of Creative Reality. You feel a fullness of mind and spirit unfettered by time and space – a feeling of knowing, of utter inclusion in the world. In your mind, you "know" your Grand Mystery is awaiting you, without question. The air is fresh, your skin is electric with feeling, your inspired life waiting to be lived.

"What's next?" you think. Then you whisper to yourself, *"Obviously!"*

Dancing in the Four Worlds

Enjoying the timeless flow of energy in the World of Creative Reality, you are filling with ideas. Listening to your inner voice of wisdom and knowledge, one answer stands above all others: "First, I want to become a masterful Alchemist!'"

As though you were waiting for magic to endorse your spirit, you look up to the heavens awaiting the god of alchemy to electrify you with a bolt of enlightenment.

"Now what's next?" you query again, testing to see if you have asked another question too soon. Looking for evidence of success, the answer to your question has already taken root. You are making notes in the soil, rapidly recording the Dance of Four Worlds, lest you forget how it works.

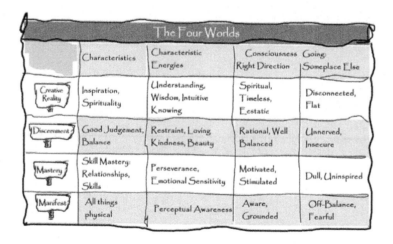

The Four Worlds				
	Characteristics	Characteristic Energies	Consciousness Going: Right Direction	Someplace Else
Creative Reality	Inspiration, Spirituality	Understanding, Wisdom, Intuitive Knowing	Spiritual, Timeless, Ecstatic	Disconnected, Flat
Discernment?	Good Judgement, Balance	Restraint, Loving Kindness, Beauty	Rational, Well Balanced	Unnerved, Insecure
Mastery	Skill Mastery: Relationships, Skills	Perseverance, Emotional Sensitivity	Motivated, Stimulated	Dull, Uninspired
Manifest?	All things physical	Perceptual Awareness	Aware, Grounded	Off-Balance, Fearful

Alchemist's Practice

Each level of our **conscious awareness** in the Four Worlds has a unique **energy**, or feeling tone. Your body, mind, spirit, and environment will manifest differently in each of the Four Worlds. It is important to tune into your senses so you may navigate the Four Worlds effectively. The practiced Alchemist of Experience becomes very adept at **sensing** and recognizing the different levels of energy in each World.

The Alchemist is keenly aware that knowledge is no substitute for experience!

1. Draw a picture of a dog standing near a stream — it doesn't need to be a perfect piece of art. Include two trees and a bush in the picture.

2. Taking a look at your *creative process* for the above drawing, describe the "energies" you experienced in your body at each level of creation.

Level of Consciousness: In the World of ...	Describe the quality of your energy in each world, e.g. fast vibration, excited, slow, agitated, muscle tension, jaw tensed.
Creative Reality	
Discernment	
Mastery	
Manifest	

∞

Chapter 11

~

Choreography

"Dance is the hidden language of the soul."
–Martha Graham

~

*"And those who were seen dancing were
thought to be insane by those who could not
hear the music."*

–Friedrich Nietzsche

Learning about the Four Worlds of consciousness and each of their energies, you have mapped what you have learned in the soil at the base of the towering Oak. Wanting to explore the vibrant energies that emanate at each level of consciousness, you become aware that you have just slid from the curiosity of Native Experience in the World of the Manifest into an anxious state in the World of Mastery. Your childlike enthusiasm to explore was quickly met with a conditioned reaction – shame. "Exploring is for children!" Those words, voiced long ago by your mother when you wanted to play instead of study, appear once more in your memory. Startled at the recognition that your consciousness changed so quickly – from excitement to shame – you conclude that there are several "features" in the Four Worlds that you hadn't anticipated and are worthy of deeper exploration! Quickly you bring your attention back to your breath and the ground beneath the Oak to regain your calm.

With this recent experience, you notice that you can alter your energies – and your consciousness – at will. You can literally move from one level to the next if, that is, you focus on the energies or state of consciousness that you would like to move into. Becoming aware of the ability to move between worlds, beneath the Oak you seat yourself in World of the Manifest where you feel grounded and alert to your Native Feelings and Thoughts. Spending time to familiarize yourself with this level, you will next venture up through each level of consciousness, one at a time, until you reach the World of Creative Reality.

Embracing first the World of the Manifest, you run your fingers through the moist soil and fallen leaves. Under the cool, leafy Oak, you experience the physical qualities of the soft and fragrant earth, the crispness of the fallen leaves, and the warm breeze tousling your hair. You think: "These are such pleasant feelings! I could surely sit here for a long time."

Ready to move on, you deliberately shift your attention to the World of Mastery. You refocus your awareness and find your emotions are like a rollercoaster. For a moment, your feelings of shame return and you begin to feel a little embarrassed at your chattering monkey mind. Suddenly, you begin to miss the Dancer! Learning the Dance of Four Worlds will clearly require some practice. It's not as easy as you thought, and sometimes you trip over your own feet. You worry that when you least expect it the Golem will grab your ankles!

Some of the time while in the World of Mastery, as you were practicing the Alchemist's skills, you were stretched beyond your comfort zone. This was a little unsettling at best, then as you got better at recognizing the energies in this level you began to feel successful – proud of yourself. The repeated practice and perseverance paid off. It felt stressful beginning to learn something new, but each time you ventured a little deeper you noticed improvement; step by step you became more familiar with your emotions and thoughts, and each time your body relaxed a little bit more. The World of Mastery was that way, too – at times stressful or frustrating, other times filled with achievement and pride. You also noticed that when you were overtired your motivation seemed to diminish to almost nothing, but when rested you were once again fully recharged and motivated.

"Becoming masterful as an Alchemist of Experience requires much learning, practice, and testing," you muse, reflecting briefly on the World of Mastery. "If I want to live into my inspired life and solve my Grand Mystery, I will need to seek experience and practice my skills." Then slipping back into the World of the Manifest, you playfully slap the ground and giggle to yourself, "That might be fun!"

Mentally, at this point noticing your consciousness hop from one world to the next you conclude, "Clearly there is a boundary between these worlds; the energies are so very different. Ah! Another 'feature!'"

Next, you deliberately elevate your consciousness up to the World of Discernment, hoping to compare the energies here to the Worlds of Mastery and the Manifest. You begin to think about why you might want to become an Alchemist, seeking to discern whether this is a choice you really do want to make. Recalling some of the problems and dilemmas you have encountered in your past, plus having experienced the joy of competence, growth, and creativity, you to begin to weigh and measure the value of this effort. Here you are able to discern the value of practicing the Alchemist's skills and can see a clear payoff for the effort. Thinking of your Grand Mystery, you know that by Dancing the Four Worlds you can add deep meaning to your own life and benefit others along the way. The World of Discernment offers considered control over the direction of your life; with reasoned logic you are able to set meaningful boundaries, make sound decisions, and stay on your journey's path.

"I like the calming energy of weighing and measuring my life's challenges," you reflect. "I am both discerning and compassionate."

With a firm finality you make a mental note, "The World of Discernment offers me safe harbor when I am seeking balance. I can regain perspective here – life has a way of sorting itself out in beautiful harmony. This is good."

With that last thought, an encompassing love fills your heart. "Yes," you think, digesting these energies, "This is indeed good."

Purposefully shifting your consciousness upward one more time you begin to daydream. You know this is the World of Creative Reality, and its quiet emptiness offers a sense of inner spaciousness. Knowing that you are fully grounded from your foundation of Core Beliefs, you begin to enjoy creative energies and discover that your ingenuity has been formed from your inner wisdom and understandings gained from your life. Space and time in this consciousness seems unimportant; the universe is your playground of inspiration and idea. You don't think this is good, you intuitively know it to be so. Life experience has taught you much, and, blending your understanding and wisdom, you feel yourself seated at the root of your own innate knowing. You have accessed the World of Creative Reality, and it is brilliant and filled with the light of inspiration. You feel lit up from inside, your intuitive knowing providing you perfect guidance. You revel in man's capacity to create according to his desire; the feelings of awe and inspiration that all humanity – and perhaps all else – is a vast communal experience existing at once and together. These impressions feel unusual at first, but you sense there is so much to explore in this world.

"Wow!" you think, gooseflesh sending out chilly tendrils of exhilaration. "Just wow!"

Without notice, and without conscious effort, the element of time and negativity once again crowd your thoughts.

"Am I too far along my life's path to begin a new undertaking? What if I want to stop – could I do it? Maybe I'll find out that I'm not a good person, and I don't want to know that! Is Dancing in the Four Worlds really a good idea? What will I do if my life changes – if I change – on the way to my Grand Mystery? Will I leave my seedlings behind?"

One question followed by another. One pro and one con at a time, you reason your way through the thick web of doubt and possibility. You sense light in your newfound darkness, inspiration in waiting.

At long last, the grey clouds of rational thought recede as the sunshine of your mind opens, allowing a single ray of thought to find purchase in the fertile ground of your intuition. You know this to be true: "This is goodness, and it's only the beginning of the Alchemist's journey!"

"I see," reflecting on your sudden decent into insecurity and your quick rise up again into discernment, "I can move up and down in the Four Worlds! Yet another 'feature.'" I've got to learn how to manage those boundaries!"

Once again in the World of Mastery, you wonder how the Dancer and her family worked so well on each of the Terraces. "That is surely a 'feature' that needs more study – once I get a little more practiced."

~

As you gain experience with the Dance of Four Worlds, the energies of each become more familiar, and you will learn to identify – in real time – which of the four worlds of consciousness you are inhabiting at any given moment. You will become adept at traveling between worlds, as you desire. Each world has its particular purpose and energetic experience. If you rise from the World of the Manifest upward, you will discover the power of self-reflection. If you move from the World of Creative Reality downward you will grasp the incredible power of your inspiration.

Perhaps you have felt victim to your own monkey mind and worked hard to sort through the variety of your emotions. Maybe you have felt like you were floating about in the Four Worlds, dancing in and out of the energies and levels of consciousness without recognizing the shifts. However, now you can see that if you simply allow your consciousness to roam on autopilot, the purpose and clarity of your journey becomes duller day by day, until it gradually diminishes into some version of "when I retire." When you are on autopilot it is enticing, if not inevitable, to believe that you are the created, not the creator. Without awareness of how you have created your world, you easily fall into the role of victim or feel that the environment is capriciously tossing you about.

In Chapter 10 we learned about ourselves from the bottom-up, from the World of the Manifest up to the World of Creative Reality. This bottom-up approach is most useful for an apprentice Alchemist just learning about your own energies; trying to gain insight into your life, solving problems or evaluating past events. We might call this style of consciousness *living into "what is"* or *reflecting on "what is."* However, bottom-up consciousness is counterproductive when we desire to *live into inspiration;* in fact, it will halt transformative inspiration in its tracks.

In this chapter, we will uncover the six basic laws and principles, or *"features,"* of Dancing in the Four Worlds. Ultimately, *living into inspiration* invites us to choreograph our dance, not simply learn the basic steps or a single dance. Living into inspiration *begins* in the World of Creative Reality and, using the *Process of Inspiration,* matures our desires until they become realized in the World of the Manifest. Living an inspired life is, indeed, a top-down initiative. It involves the creative use of all that we have learned as Alchemists of Experience and invites us to live playfully in a world chock-full of possibility.

Certainly, there will times of confusion, dilemmas, fear, and disappointing results. You may take one step forward, and two back; at other times you will be able to launch yourself forward into transformative growth. This is, after all, real life. However, with sufficient practice and perseverance, you will make great strides forward. Returning to automatic pilot and getting covered with sludge in The Bog will no longer be enticing or long-lasting; now you know how to get back on the Paths of Wellness and Inspiration, tend your Alchemist's Garden, and dance up *and* down the Terraces of consciousness in each of the Four Worlds.

Embrace the incredible power of your own inspiration, all that it means to be *you*. Clarity of consciousness in the Four Worlds provides deep footing and strength of purpose for actualizing your inspiration. Not only will we do the Dance of Four Worlds, but we will become the choreographers of our own lives, of our own dance.

First Dance

Materializing as if from nowhere — sitting in your Alchemist's Garden, admiring your seedlings — you hear someone murmur, "How can I help you?"

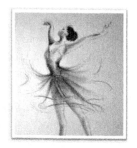

Looking up at once, the Dancer sits before you, looking quite pleased with herself.

"What do you mean?" you whisper with muted astonishment.

"When the student is ready...," she begins.

"The teacher will appear," you conclude.

An uncomfortable silence seats itself between you and the Dancer. Smoothing the dirt and stacking the dried leaves, as if clearing the debris between you, you decide to confide a bit about yourself.

"I have a Grand Mystery," you confess softly as though some unknown Golem were listening in insidious preparation. "I want to understand how relationships work."

"Good," says the Dancer, "You are starting at the beginning, just where you should start! The magic of creation starts precisely here."

A lengthy silence once again takes up accommodation between you as you self-consciously reorganize the soil and stack the drying leaves.

"Please, don't wait for me," the Dancer says.

"Well, what's next?" you demand.

"Precisely!" congratulates the Dancer. "Well done!"

Stillness once again descends; more reorganizing the dry leaves.

"Well, I am ready," you say, "...and you are the teacher, yes? Like I said, what's next?!"

In the moment's discomfort you begin to reflect: "Well, if I never have a relationship then I know I will never know how one works. On the other hand, if I risk practice and learn about them I know I will eventually find a companion...."

In your mind's eye, you can see the vague silhouette of your future sojourner.

Concluding aloud to the Dancer, "If I want to have a relationship then I need to find someone to have one with."

"This is a fine discernment!" says the Dancer, revealing her quiet smile and warm heart.

"But only you are here with me."

"Ah," says the Dancer, "Evidence of Success!"

The angst of the Dancer's cryptic responses is beginning to wear on your inspiration. "Don't be tart with me!" shoot the words of frustration from your mouth.

And with that the Dancer vanishes in a misty wisp.

~

The steps toward living into inspiration are simple; however, as novice Alchemists we usually stumble into the potholes of inexperience with great surprise. As a heads-up, let's look at the

Laws and Principles governing the Dance of Four Worlds, and illustrate one or two potholes we might encounter on our journey.

It is law – Each of the Four Worlds has a unique purpose. The *Principle of Consciousness* asserts that each level of consciousness has a specific purpose.

The first step is getting a foothold on your Grand Mystery in the World of Creative Reality. It begins with acknowledging a deep personal yearning; a longing melancholy that resides in near silence deep within your heart. Your yearnings are not just today's needs, but lifelong desires you deeply want to realize. What do you yearn for in your own life and for each of your seedlings? This is the time to listen to the one deep inside and allow your yearnings to share their compassionate voice.

Discernment invites you to weigh and balance your alternatives. The purpose of consciousness in the World of Discernment is to clarify value and define boundaries.

The World of Mastery summons you to master your interpersonal skills and know-how. This is one of the most difficult of worlds to master, and our own emotional patterning and that of others can be quite complex and challenging to master.

Purpose in the World of the Manifest is to complete a Quest and share your results out into the physical world. The Manifest world is filled with giving forth our own creations and receiving the creations of others. It is glorious to spend time in this completed state of affairs.

Remember that you are the creator, not the created. So often, we stop our efforts at yearning and impatiently await evidence of completion. "Ask, and you shall receive," we chant to ourselves, as though someone were going to present it to us – completed – in some priestly "since-you-have-asked" fashion. It doesn't work like that; you must create your own movement, your own forward momentum. Moving from desire to manifested reality requires that you frequently ask, "What's next?" Then, discern and balance your alternatives, "do," and execute what needs to be done before basking in what you have created.

Each world has its unique purpose; therefore, your moves must be purposeful.

It is law – Creation is iterative. The *Principle of Movement* between and within worlds is crucial in shaping our outcomes.

Creating the life you yearn for requires that you continuously shape and refine your inspiration in each of the Four Worlds in order to have it materialize. Turning desire into reality is usually an iterative experience as you move from one world to another to adjust your ideas, respond to lessons learned, evaluate their merits, learn more about what is needed, and continue to build until your results are what you have envisioned.

Iterative creation requires that you move between worlds, for example, one day imagining in the World of Creation, then the next discerning your alternatives. You may then return to Creative Reality to imagine a little deeper, then go directly to Mastery to test out an idea. Movement is rarely straightforward from one world to the next, but varies depending on what is needed: "What's next?"

Movement within worlds calls you to balance our energies, as in a recipe. Perhaps, for example, in the World of Creative Reality you need a little more understanding to round out your wisdom, or maybe you need to shift your energies for a stronger blend of wisdom to validate your intuitive knowing. In the World of Mastery you might work to balance your strength and drive with a bit of empathy and compromise. Each world asks you to balance its energies to accomplish the task at hand.

Finally, movement within the worlds often requires us to create a mixture of energies between worlds. For example, in judging the rude behavior of an individual it might be important to combine your intuition in the World of Creation with a balanced sense of discernment – compassion and judgment – before any conclusions are made.

Sometimes our feelings, emotions, and thoughts can become either too rigid or too chaotic. If we become rigidly dominant in the World of Mastery, for example, we may lose our sense of compassion and fail to discern reasoned decision-making for our families or for the greater good. Or imagine if we hopped from one world, or one energy, randomly to another; decision-making would be confused, actions would be non-purposeful, and our effectiveness would be lost. Good Alchemy requires that we move between worlds and within energies with knowledge and self-awareness.

The Principle of Movement in Iterative Creation comes with the responsibility to move with conscious awareness.

It is law – All questions have an answer. The *Principle of Dual Nature* asserts that within our singular selves we have both our observer and the selves we observe working together without error.

In our day-to-day lives we become embroiled in our personal journeys; we travel between worlds and dance with our energies as we pursue our Grand Mystery. But we all know how easy it is to feel stuck in our movement, or chaotic in our dance. Our dual nature, having our observed, everyday selves, and our deeper knowing of our aware self provides us with both the actor and our guidance system. Wherever and whenever we need assistance we need only ask our deepest awareness, "What's Next?" or any other question for that matter. All questions have an answer from our always-loving deeper selves. Our dual nature works in perfect harmony within us, always available for reliable awareness, intuitive knowing, and perfect guidance. We need only ask!

Asking, "What's next?" allows us to stay the course on the journey to our Grand Mystery (precisely!). In the timeless world of imagination and inspiration, in the World of Creative Reality, an answer in the form of a feeling, or a visualization, a thought or an urge will let you know what is next. If your questions are not answered, you are not yet a skilled listener. The practice of "Emptying the vessel and then listening" is a critical skill. The answer will be there; perhaps an image will trigger a thought or a feeling. Something in your environment may give you an idea, but you must learn to listen. It is a practice; marinate in your question for a moment, a day or a week! The answer will be there because the question has been asked – there are no exceptions.

It is law – Boundaries divide adjacent worlds. The *Principle of Permeability* asserts there is an optimal flow between levels of consciousness.

Between each of the Four Worlds there is a virtual boundary. The inspired, timeless energies in World of Creative Reality, for example, are very different from the judging, balancing, and discerning energies in the World of Discernment. By the same token, the energies of Discernment are very different than the reactive, conditioned emotions – even the joy of persistence and success – in the World of Mastery. Each of the Four Worlds has a defining purpose held in place by a boundary.

The Principle of Permeability allows us to move between worlds, but the boundaries, too, have the characteristics of rigidity or chaos. If a boundary becomes too rigid, the world adjacent to it becomes inaccessible. For example, imagine a person that is considered a psychopath – one that can hurt others without a sense of guilt. For these individuals, their world of emotion is utterly divorced from their sense of right or wrong, making any desired action a good one without moral consequence. On the other hand, if a boundary between worlds becomes too permeable, it is easy to lose direction or to lack purpose; our inspiration gets easily diluted or redirected elsewhere.

Unique to this law, boundaries between worlds can also overlap one another outside of our awareness. Overlapping boundaries are a significant cause of confused thinking, emotions, and reactions.

There are many situations in real life that can challenge our boundaries; this is where life can get difficult if we have debris in our path. Look at an example where we may question or doubt our desires, for instance, by asking, "Do I really want a relationship?" and then declaring, "I'm not that good at them anyway." Or someone else may challenge our decisions or point of view.

Examining this example, once a challenge is initiated, then the angel and devil, sitting on opposite shoulders, begin to debate and discern. The purpose here is to ask challenging questions, seeking decisions that resonate deeply within ourselves and are in alignment with our Grand Mystery. We find balance and equanimity in our thought and feelings. In many cases, discernment is relatively straightforward with only periodic rebalancing being necessary – our boundaries are properly permeable.

In many other cases, however, conditioned emotions from the World of Mastery intrude on our logic. This confusion is problematic, in that conditioned emotions are inappropriately seeping into the World of Discernment. Practice in recognizing your state of consciousness in each of the Four Worlds is absolutely necessary. Mastering the distinctions, or boundaries, between worlds can make or break an inspiration wending its way into the world.

Maureen, a single woman who deeply desired a life partner, knew she needed to meet someone to begin a relationship. Her idea of a "relationship" seedling was straightforward; however, when she entered the World of Discernment she questioned her desire. Was this what she really wanted? At this juncture, her thinking became a little clouded:

> *Maureen: I want a relationship, and I need to find a person to have a relationship with – at least for starters. A good relationship is a healthy part of life, but most potential partners my age are so screwed up I don't think I'll ever find one!*

The first part of her inspiration was clear and straightforward. She yearned for a relationship and owned that it was up to her to begin one. However, years of picking "troubled" partners and experiencing little success tinted her logical thinking with emotional debris. This was a difficult and confusing area for Maureen to navigate.

For Maureen, inspiration and discernment were in full operation, but the boundary between the World of Discernment and the World of Mastery was fuzzy. She was unable to tell when her conditioned thinking and emotions colored her logic. From her point of view, she could never get what she wanted – a self-fulfilling reality. Maureen didn't recognize she was going in the wrong direction.

Were Maureen to better understand the distinction between the World of Discernment and the World of Mastery, she might have considered one or more of the following actions.

She might reflect back on her last relationship and determine how she might better discern between a "troubled" versus an "emotionally healthy" person. What would be characteristics and indicators of emotional well-being?

She may listen to her friend, using the Alchemist's Language to see if (s)he were going in the right direction, or somewhere else.

Reflecting back on her last relationship, she might use the Alchemist's Language to see what her own language and self-talk revealed. She could now begin to move her language in the "right direction."

If she uncovered conditioned emotional thinking blocking her path forward, she could use the Debris Wiper to clear the way.

When with a new person, she might practice tuning into her here-and-now Native Experience. This would give her a cleaner, more direct experience of this new friend rather than filtering her reactions through conditioned emotion. Native feelings are trustworthy – listen to your gut.

Check to see if her patterns of choosing "troubled" partners indicated the presence of her Golem. Perhaps she was unconsciously living into her mythology from early life experiences – some version of "You don't deserve a good partner."

Practice the energies of the World of Discernment and the World of Mastery, separately, so she could more readily identify when her boundaries were getting hazy; when emotion was coloring discernment.

Brainstorming sessions are another excellent example to explore what happens when a boundary becomes clouded or too porous, and competing energies combine and cause difficulty and confusion. Consider what happens when the boundary between the World of Creative Reality and the World of Discernment become clouded. Remember a time when you have participated in a brainstorming session. The facilitator usually begins by instructing participants to listen to suggestions non-judgmentally, noting that the purpose of brainstorming is to generate ideas without judging them when they arise. In essence, the facilitator is attempting to generate ideas and inspiration from the World of Creative Reality.

What often happens after a couple of ideas are generated, however, is that someone will rain on the parade by declaring, "That idea won't work because...(fill in the blank)." At that point, the discussion either gets diverted to address the criticism or the facilitator will intervene.

What's happening? Looking at the interaction from the Four Worlds of consciousness, the expansive energies of timelessness, of ideas and inspiration are suddenly bombarded by the constraining energies of discernment, of weighing and measuring alternatives. You may have noticed how the positive energy of the brainstorm gets thwarted by the shift in consciousness and its purpose. Notice how the flow of ideas comes to a crashing halt, your muscles tighten, and you look toward the facilitator for help. You can feel the energies clash leaving dissatisfaction and conflict in its wake. These are not disagreements, they are a collision of energies each well intended yet having a different purpose.

As you begin to practice the Alchemy of Experience, remain watchful. Ask, "What's next?" and listen to your answer emerging from within. Discern your choices carefully without clouding or overlapping the boundaries from other levels of consciousness. Practice and master your budding Alchemist's skills; there will be ups and downs, and eventual success as you persevere.

~

Second Dance

Rejoining with your thoughts about the Dancer's disappearance you wonder, "Where did the Dancer go? She simply vanished as mysteriously as she appeared?"

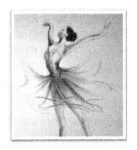

A gnarly compression grips your chest as you notice the sudden loss of companionship.

"Well, I'm not the best person with relationships," you acknowledge. "Maybe I should have considered her comment to better discern what she meant to say. After all, she was there when I told her I had no one," you recalled.

"I'm sorry," you whisper apologetically in the Dancer's absence. "You were the Evidence of Success the whole while!"

"Exactly!" murmured the Dancer re-appearing just as strangely as she vanished. "You have mastered something new!"

Slipping into Native Joy, a warm smile extends itself upward toward your heart.

~

It is law – Progress is a constant. The *Principle of Evidence of Success* asserts that life always moves in the direction of your alignment.

Often in the Process of Creation we "Ask and Then Listen." We discern the issues that lie in our paths and then become conscientious in the World of Mastery by "doing" and "building" the lives we yearn for. Often, we can easily see the results of our creative process; Evidence of Success stands tall in our line of sight. For example, if I set out to write a poem, the completed poem is obvious evidence.

Sometimes, however, Evidence of Success is not so easily recognized. We have all had times when it feels like we are pushing the boulder – a creative project – uphill only to have it tumble back down to where we began. Experience like this lets us know that we don't know how to "Look for Evidence of Success" in that situation. However, the evidence is there if we learn how to look by challenging our mythologies, changing our perspective, or looking for progress in new places.

In the years following my divorce I yearned once again for an intimate relationship. My mother, worrying about her discouraged daughter, set me up with the handsome son of her best friend. He had a touch of ADHD (more than a touch) and was not appealing to me as a love interest, but we became fast friends. He was great fun and always full of adventure. Every time I needed a friend, he was there. Every time I wanted to share something about my son – or my work – he was there. If I became forlorn, he was there. If I was bored, he was there.

Then a miracle happened. It was as if a great, slow churning gear shifted in my inner knowing, a piece of debris clogging my inner vision fell to the ground, and a new panorama came into view; I experienced a change of perspective, and before my eyes someone I was in love with stood at the foot of my yearning. My dear friend, soon to be my lover, appeared before me – somehow changed. My Evidence of Success had been in clear view all the while, although my view had been clouded by undeciphered debris, conditioned emotion.

Those times when Evidence of Success seems elusive we need to learn how to look for it, to see past our mythologies and predisposed thinking and look beyond, or on the periphery, of where we ordinarily place our gaze. Sometimes we need to look with our feelings and not our eyes, or listen with our intuition instead of our ears. Consider rearranging the puzzle pieces of your life and gain fresh perspective. We need to keep all of our senses, our hearts and our minds, trained on our Grand Mystery.

When Evidence of Success is in clear view, consider yourself fortunate. More often, however, your evidence lies within a new understanding or a fresh perspective on your point of view. It doesn't work to look for Evidence of Success in what you lack or while you are engaged in distraction; and you surely won't find it if you are going someplace else wrapped in negativity, as here all things are flawed.

Paraphrasing Dorothy in the Wizard of Oz, "Home was there all the time, I just didn't see it." For the budding Alchemist, "ask and you will hear, look and you will see."

It is Law – The *Principle of Community* asserts that a community creates itself through the consciousness of its individual participants.

Communities are made up of two or more individuals, each bringing to the group their individual Grand Mysteries, their varied mix of energies and unique dances in the Four Worlds. Communities contain the potential for powerful contribution and membership, and they can flounder together in disorganization.

The Principle of Community asserts that communities create themselves through individuals co-creating with others within the group. In a simple example, when a group of people are working to "get out the vote" during an election, a small community will be formed to call registered voters and remind them to come out on Election Day. If each individual in the small group were focused in the World of Mastery, a cohesive community effort would be underway to achieve positive results.

If, on the other hand, that same small group of people were called together to make voter calls, and half the people were debating whether it would be better to make calls or come up with a more effective strategy, the group would become disorganized. Becoming divided, half the individuals would be working in the World of Mastery, making the required calls and focusing on completing their task. The other half of the group would be debating get-out-the-vote strategies and their merits in the World of Discernment. Imagine the interpersonal dynamics that might result from leaving this group disorganized and contentious.

There are many ways in which communities create themselves and evolve. As with our individual journeys, self-awareness is critical in navigating our way to our Grand Mystery. So, too, communities of people must be knowledgeable about the group's Grand Mystery, its desired contribution, and how each individuals' participation supports alignment with the community's direction or is going someplace else.

~

Third Dance

Continuing to chat with the Dancer, the two of you begin to discuss how to tend the Alchemist's Garden.

"Tending my seedlings is my greatest joy," the Dancer confesses as she draws her hands to her heart. "All that I deeply love flourishes when I cultivate them thoughtfully. I prune their withering leaves, remove caked-on debris that stunts their growth and nourish them with acceptance and encouragement."

"How can I nourish my 'relationship' seedling?" you ask, feeling as though your discouraged heart has just been squeezed through a sieve.

"Ah," nods the understanding Dancer, "Nourish yourself with self-compassion and love. Honor your seedlings with the same. You'll see, they will grow strong and able, as will you."

After rearranging the remaining spattering of dried leaves between you, you draw your hands to your heart and feel their warm embrace.

"Thank you," you mumble into your chest as the Dancer's loving energy coats your spirit.

"What's next?" you ask yourself gazing at your seedling packets. *"It's time to plant you, I know what you are."*

To share this heartfelt success, you look up expectantly to see only a hand-spade where the Dancer had been sitting.

"Precisely!" you think, *"Evidence of Success."*

From the top Terrace, the Dancer, again reunited with her family, bows a quiet *Namaste*.

You blow a kiss in silent appreciation: "Thank you."

~

The Choreography of Inspiration

Practicing the Dance of Four Worlds will open up new worlds of experience as you dive into the energies of each level of consciousness and become more familiar with their territory. There are governing laws and supporting principles for Dancing in the Four Worlds. Over time you will become more confident in your skills and move between and within worlds with ease. The journey to your Grand Mystery is filled with many Quests, unexpected adventures, and surprises along the way. As you learn the Dance of Four Worlds and move on to more advanced skills, you will become adept at living into your inspiration and knowing that you are the creator of your own life experience at each step and for every dance.

Unfortunately, life never rolls out the turf before us in any step-wise fashion. If we live on autopilot we will surely weave in and out of the

Terraces until we are dropped back off in The Bog in utter frustration. However, we can learn to choreograph our steps, create our own dance, and move with inspired improvisation as we dance our treasured contributions out from inspiration and onto the stage of our own lives.

Choreography is the composition and arrangement of our dances in the Four Worlds. Once we learn the steps and the basic dance, we may choose to change up our footing, speed the pace, or rearrange the dance itself. We may create our own unique dances when inspired to do so. The Alchemist, mastering the laws and principles of the Four Worlds, must learn the Choreography of Inspiration.

The six fundamental laws and corresponding principles for Dancing in the Four Worlds are more concisely summarized below. As long as you are mindful of these principles, you will dance with clarity and cultivate the Alchemist's art form, the choreography of inspiration. Forgetting these principles will lead your dance astray, your thinking will become sloppy, and your results may not be what you had hoped for. Understanding the Laws and Principles of the Four Worlds will give you wisdom and understanding as you live into your inspired life.

Law #1 – Each World Has a Unique Purpose – The Principle of Consciousness asserts that our states of consciousness shift to achieve the purpose of each world.

Each world has its own unique purpose that is different from the other worlds.

The World of Creative Reality connects us to the Source of all the energies in our universe and enables receptiveness to our own spiritual experience. This consciousness includes the energies of inspiration, wisdom, understanding, and intuitive knowing.

The World of Discernment focuses our consciousness on critical thinking and decision-making allowing us to discern our values and make choices, and to form boundaries as we arrive at "right thinking," the harmonious balance between compassion and control.

Discernment consciousness includes the energies of unconditional love, restraint, and harmony when balance is achieved.

The World of Mastery enables us to build our skills, whether they be emotional development, interpersonal, or professional skills. The energies of dominance, perseverance, and empathy characterize this level of consciousness as we seek balance in the relationship sphere on this level.

The World of Manifestation allows us to be grounded in physical reality, to navigate our inspiration to completion in our lives day-to-day: at work, driving a car, raising our children, or simply cleaning our house. The energies of consciousness include completion, release, the satisfaction of giving, and the appreciation of receiving.

Our state of consciousness and its corresponding energies will vary in accordance of the purpose of each world.

Law #2 – Creation Is Iterative – The Principle of Movement asserts that we are free to move within a single world's energies, or between the Four Worlds in any order we choose.

It is not necessary to move sequentially from top to bottom, or from bottom to top in the Four Worlds. We may begin a Quest in the World of Creative Reality and hop immediately into the World of Mastery. We may begin a Quest in the World of Manifestation and move into Discernment where we evaluate the merits of something newly created.

Navigating the Four Worlds can occur from bottom-to-top (beginning in the World of the Manifest), or from top-to-bottom (beginning in the World of Creative Reality).

Bottom-to-top navigation usually implies a process of *self-reflection*; that is, looking at what has been manifested (either physically, emotionally, or logically) and understanding how it occurred.

Top-to-bottom navigation employs the process of *inspiration and creation*; starting with an inspired idea and evolving it through the

Four Worlds until it becomes realized, or manifested.

We may also choose to combine the energies in one world with the energies in another, such as being angry at someone while also experiencing love and compassion, or intuitively sensing the direction of a relationship and establishing boundaries to protect our values.

There are no limits on the number of permutations and combinations available to us in the Four Worlds.

Realizing our inspiration is an iterative process. We may move in and out of worlds and states of consciousness many times in order to reach our intended outcomes.

Law #3 – All Questions Have an Answer – The Principle of Dual Nature asserts that our observer and the selves we observe work together without error.

All questions have an answer. Our dual natures, our two-sided nature of being both observer and the observed, allows us to ask any question with our observer able to provide an answer. All questions are answered, no exceptions.

Law #4 – Each World Has Its Boundaries – The Principle of Permeability asserts that boundaries between worlds must be permeable to achieve well-being.

Each world has an invisible boundary between the world above it and the next lower world. In state of well-being, the boundaries are clear, yet permeable. Energies in one world will interact with those in another as balance is achieved and inspiration is manifested.

For example, if you are experiencing a strong reaction in the emotional World of Mastery, say anger, you may choose to reflect on the usefulness of the emotion, or the behavior it produces, in the World of Discernment. There you may elect to control your emotional behavior and provide yourself some self-compassion.

Boundaries between worlds can be healthy (permeable), or maladaptive (rigid, undefined, or overlapping). Poorly defined boundaries can produce sloppy thinking and poor results, can limit your well-being, or can send you in a direction going somewhere else.

For example, an individual with a fully rigid boundary between the World of Mastery and the World of Discernment may be impulsive and lack compassion and good judgment. Alternatively, the person may be extremely logical and unaware of their feelings or emotions.

Law #5 – Progress Is Constant – The Principle of Evidence of Success asserts that progress is always present in the direction you have chosen.

Progress is a constant in the direction you have chosen. You choose to move in the direction of your well-being, choose to move in the direction away from your well-being, or choose not to move at all and reverse your momentum through atrophy. There is always Evidence of Success that is in alignment with the direction of travel.

If you are aligned in the direction of your Grand Mystery and your Quests, you will find Evidence of Success even in the smallest of steps.

If you are headed in a negative direction, you will find Evidence of Success in the negative direction. (Success toward a negative destination indicates that you are not acting in your best interests.)

If you are not moving forward (in other words, standing still), momentum will deteriorate and eventually reverse its direction

Law #6 – Communities Are a Shared Creation – The Principle of Community asserts that communities create themselves through the consciousness of its individual participants.

Two or more people comprise a "community" where individuals are engaged in a common activity. The Principle of Community asserts that each individual operates from their unique Four Worlds consciousness. Together the community will act either synergistically, in conflict, or independently.

Synergistic communities share the same level of consciousness; for example, all members are focused in the World of Discernment and are applying sound reasoning to evaluate an outcome.

Conflict arises in communities that are unknowingly operating at different levels of consciousness; for example, one individual is acting from the world of emotion (the World of Mastery) and another is operating judgmentally (the World of Discernment).

Four Worlds Laws and Principles	
#1 Each of the Four Worlds has a unique purpose.	The Principle of Consciousness asserts that each state of consciousness has a purpose.
#2 Creation is iterative.	The Principle of Movement asserts that movement between and within worlds is crucial in shaping our outcomes.
#3 All questions are answered.	The Principle of Dual Nature asserts that our observer and the selves we observe work together without error.
#4 There are boundaries between worlds.	The principle of Permeability asserts there is an optimal balance between levels of consciousness.
#5 There is always evidence of success.	The Principle of Progress asserts that there is always evidence of progress in the direction of your alignment.
#6 Community is a shared creation.	The Principle of Community asserts that communities create themselves through combined consciousness of its individuals.

Independently functioning groups in a community co-exist together without impacting each other; for example, in an organization where the Legal department functions primarily in the World of Discernment weighing the merits of its cases, while a Product Development group strives for innovation in the World of Creative Reality.

Living into inspiration is an individually choreographed Dance through each of the Four Worlds. Understanding the Laws and Principles of the Four Worlds enables you to move between each purposeful world in accordance with what comes next along your journey. Each state of consciousness enables you to access and balance your energies as you apply wisdom, understanding, discernment, and skill to realize your desires.

Creating your inspired life requires that you shape and mold each of your results to perfection. Fully living into inspiration is an iterative process with many baby steps, successes, and failures along the way – all are parts of the journey on the way to your Grand Mystery. Evidence of Success is available to you at each step along the path – simply pause and acknowledge your progress.

As a budding Alchemist, practice Dancing in the Four Worlds: innovate the steps of each dance, and choreograph the arrangement of your art form. By now you know the steps, and you have all the tools. There is nothing left to do but dance audaciously into your inspired life.

~

Finale

Becoming more at ease with the Dance of Four Worlds, you drift into reverie and begin to imagine your own Choreography in the Four Worlds. In your mind, you hear the beat of your own drummer – your own inspiration – and you begin to dance.

First, reaching your hands upward to the sky, you draw back in a rich array of energies from source feeding your wisdom, understanding, and your deepest knowing from all that is – at least, as much as you can manage for now. As you draw in energy, you feel the urge to sway, and then twist gently right, then left and back again. Once more you reach to the sky and spread your arms wide, as though offering appreciation, "Yes, this is right!" – a smile crosses your lips.

Next, you hop back a step as if surprised and begin to dust off imagined debris from your clothes; "I'm done with those old emotions!" you assert, and begin to smooth out the cloth along your arms and legs. "From now on I am going to seek balance and harmony!"

Finally, you kneel to the earth, relishing its fragrance and cool feel on your fingertips. "Ah," you murmur, "this is good!"

Unexpectedly, you begin to feel a little silly laying on the ground; embarrassed actually. You remember how you were teased when you were younger for dancing alone, especially if you were doing unusual movements.

Reaching up to discern these sour feelings in your consciousness, you take note of how untrue your dancing myth really is: you can dance alone or in a community, and unusual steps are a sign of creativity. You are actually inspired to move as you are. Feeling a flood of self-compassion, you drift once again into movement and enjoy the rewards of perseverance, of "hanging in there" and continuing your practice.

After some time, your movements begin to feel a little stale; you are becoming bored. "I know," you think, "I must be done with this dance!" Dance manifested and complete! You can sense the Dancer's distant appreciation of your practice.

Astutely you move right into to the "Big Question": "What's next?"

A few moments go by, your mind comfortably calm, empty, and receptive as the answer surfaces into your quiet state of mind.

"I'll write a Thank-You note to the Dancer!" you think sentimentally, "She has given me the goodness of Dance."

From the very crown of your head, settling into your intuitive heart, you hear the Dancer silently murmur, "You're welcome!"

~

Four Worlds Choreography

Inspiration

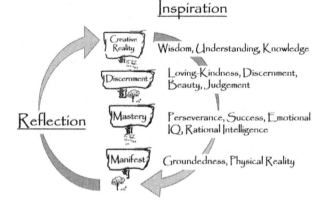

Reflection

Creative Reality — Wisdom, Understanding, Knowledge

Discernment — Loving-Kindness, Discernment, Beauty, Judgement

Mastery — Perseverance, Success, Emotional IQ, Rational Intelligence

Manifest — Groundedness, Physical Reality

Alchemist's Practice

Four Worlds Laws and Principles	
#1 Each of the Four Worlds has a unique purpose.	The Principle of Consciousness asserts that each state of consciousness has a purpose.
#2 Creation is iterative.	The Principle of Movement asserts that movement between and within worlds is crucial in shaping our outcomes.
#3 All questions are answered.	The Principle of Dual Nature asserts that our observer and the selves we observe work together without error.
#4 There are boundaries between worlds.	The principle of Permeability asserts there is an optimal balance between levels of consciousness.
#5 There is always evidence of success.	The Principle of Progress asserts that there is always evidence of progress in the direction of your alignment.
#6 Community is a shared creation.	The Principle of Community asserts that communities create themselves through combined consciousness of its individuals.

Living into inspiration is a **choregraphed Dance** – from **top to bottom** and from **bottom to top** – through each of the Four Worlds. Understanding the **Laws and Principles** of the Four Worlds enables you to move between each purposeful world in accordance with **what comes next** along your journey. The master Alchemist understands the laws and principles, has tested them all and practiced them hundreds of times over.

1. Reflect back on the drawing of the tree by the stream you completed in Chapter 10 – or think of a recent experience where you used your creative process.

Recent Experience

_____

_____

_____

_____

_____

2. Make notes below on how you may have experienced each of the *Four Worlds Laws and Principles*. You may only notice a few of the laws or principles in action on your first try.

Practice often!

Four Worlds Law and Principles		
#1	Each of the Four Worlds has a unique purpose.	The principle of consciousness asserts that our states of consciousness shift to achieve the purpose of each world.
Notes		
#2	Creation is iteractive.	The principle of Movement asserts that movement between and withing worlds is crucial in shaping our outcomes.
Notes		
#3	All questions are answered.	The principle of Dual Nature asserts that our observer and the selves we observe work together without error.
Notes		
#4	There are boundaries between worlds.	The principle of Permeability asserts there is an optimal balance between levels of consciousness.
Notes		
#5	There is always evidence of success.	The principle of Progress asserts that there is always evidence of progress in the direction of your alignment.
Notes		
#6	Community is a shared creation.	The principle of Community asserts that communities create themselves through combined consciousness of its individuals.
Notes		

∞

Chapter 12

~

And in the End

*"It would...be a beautiful thing to pass through
life together hypnotized in our dreams: your
dream for your country; our dream for humanity;
our dream for science."*

–Pierre Curie's marriage proposal to Madame
Marie Sklodowska Curie

~

*"If I see anything vital around me, it is
precisely that spirit of adventure, which seems
indestructible and is akin to curiosity."*

–Madame Marie Sklodowska Curie

Sitting by a small pond bordering your garden, you become
ensconced in the sweet nectar of life brimming with potential, you
imagine you could see right over the horizon to the foothills of your
Grand Mystery and the Treasure that awaits. But it's just a hair's
breadth beyond your reach.

In your newly gained wisdom you close your eyes, settle into the empty quiet of your mind, and ask, "What's next?"

~

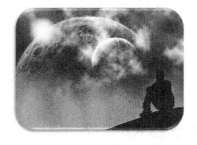

For the Alchemist of Experience, traveling through the Quagmire is a Frontier Adventure of the very best kind. The exquisite hills and valleys are teeming with life and offer many unexpected thrills and challenges. There is always new territory to explore and so much to learn about ourselves and those around us. The Alchemist is never bored – unless, that is, a rest is needed – and has the innate ability to create the life that is deeply yearned for.

Living into your inspired life is an ongoing journey. There is always more that lies ahead, and the adventure is never done. There are plenty of twists and turns along way, and if you choose a route that you don't particularly favor, you can always change your mind, mid-course correct, and resume your travels in the right direction. One must always be alert, however, to recognize distractions as unproductive detours and learn to have compassion for your Golem; it is only a lonely, fictitious creature that wants to be put to bed.

In our final chapter, our travels together as author and reader will come to an end. It is my deepest desire, however, to send you off with a freshly packed Alchemist's Knapsack. It will contain three things:

   ✓ A reminder of the raw materials you have at your fingertips to navigate the continuing journey

   ✓ A map of the territory

   ✓ A Guidebook containing the processes, laws, and principles the Alchemist of Experience abides by

Opening the Alchemist's Knapsack

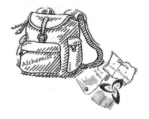

The Amulet

Reaching into your Alchemist's Knapsack, the first thing you extract is an amulet, a charm that has three intersecting loops with a jasmine center. The letters SMBE are inscribed, one in each of the four shapes. The letter "S" is centered in the green jasmine stone.

Why do we have this amulet? The amulet represents the raw materials with which we travel through the Quagmire. The delicate jasmine center containing the letter "S" is represents your spiritual center; this is the knower, or deep internal "awareness," that answers our most challenging questions. It is the essence of who we are. Our knowing self is always in communion with all that is around us and within us. Our self, or spirit, is a valuable participant in the universal experience we share with all other people, animals, and the environment. We are "all-knowing" in that we know what we do know, and we know what we don't know. We also have the ability and freedom of choice to educate ourselves further in whatever way we desire.

Within our deepest selves, we have our Core Beliefs to ground us in the Quagmire. Knowing who we are, and holding ourselves in high esteem, we will always be communicating with integrity and seeing the same in others. Leaders unto ourselves we stop, look, and listen to the world around us, knowing that wisdom and personal leadership are imperative. We know when to surrender, as not all battles are won through might. Finally, valuing our well-being, we understand that we always have the choice to go in the *right direction* for ourselves – or not, which is also a choice. Always righting ourselves on our Quests, we practice "non-harming" and walk away from ignorance. Ignorance may have a pretty package, but its contents hold no value.

In the top loop of the amulet is an "M" that represents the power of our minds. Our Minds are our training ground in life and provide us valuable information that is sometimes true, and other times false and outdated. Our emotional baggage from previous experiences lives in our minds, and we have the power to challenge our outdated logic and personal mythologies. Our ability to learn and our powerful intellects continuously inform us of our alternatives and help us reason, weigh, and measure possible outcomes.

Although the truth of our innate selfhood – *that we are creators of our own lives* – is known to our spirit, our minds serve to refresh our thinking so we may make better choices on the journey toward our own Grand Mystery.

Ego lives in our minds along with our memories, thoughts, emotions, myths, and scripts. Our minds, or egos, love to think they are the masters of our seafaring souls, but our spirit is the true navigator. The ego asks its questions; spirit answers.

The left loop of the amulet holds a "B" to remind us of our body: its native strength, health, and well-being. Our bodies are a tremendous resource housing our endurance, flexibility, and resilience. We often take our wellness for granted, especially when have no physical ailments. However, how we choose to maintain ourselves begins to show as we grow older. Unreleased stress and emotion, inactivity, poor diet, and insufficient sleep will eventually take its toll on our health and detour us on a journey to *someplace else*, which is not a desirable destination! Many conditions are reversible, and in all situations it is possible to choose to travel in the direction of well-being. We choose each step, each path, and ultimately, the ease of our journey.

The "E" in the left loop of the amulet represents our environment. Clearly, toxic environments polluted with chemicals, exhaust, preservatives, and other poisons are lethal to our mental, physical, and spiritual well-being. Also included in the arena of environment are our home, work, and other personal spaces. Cluttered and dirty spaces create stress, as do people that introduce toxic personalities – or energies – into our lives.

On the other hand, environments that introduce beauty – to each his or her own! – have the power to release stress, increase our feelings of pleasure, and can provide our bodies, minds, and spirit with a healthy haven in which to thrive.

Our bodies, minds, spirit, and environment are all integrated; one impacts upon the other, either for the better or by dragging us backward to *someplace else*. A poor night's sleep, for example, will slow our thinking the next day; a good run can enhance our creativity; breathing in cigarette smoke can kill us.

The Alchemist's Amulet is a token to remind us of the raw materials of "us" as we journey to our Grand Mystery. The better our choices about actively *living into our well-being* as we go in the *right direction*, the greater health and vitality we will enjoy – along with a longer lifespan.

It is your choice – every minute of every day – to *live fully into the life you yearn for*. By embracing your Core Beliefs, you possess the raw materials of your journey.

Map of the Territory

The Map of the Quagmire, the territory through which you travel, has many paths to follow. Not all paths are productive, and many can lead you to places you don't want to go. However, several are of high value and some routes are less traveled. Each path will get you to the next succeeding trailhead and prepare you for its unique experience.

Starting your journey on the Path of Wellness, you learn to identify your body, mind, spirit, and environment and come to understand the attributes of well-being for each. It is on the Path of Wellness that you learn to discern each individual aspect of yourself, then practice integrating them together to learn about how you work in totality. Each aspect of *you* – body, mind, spirit, and environment – must be clearly understood in its individual parts before you can fruitfully understand how to use them together.

It is so easy to clump our "well-being" into saying a single "Oh, I'm good" or "Um, I'm not so good," but without clear distinctions about our four aspects, we often quite inadvertently head someplace else. It is like trying to row a canoe in a straight line from point A to point B with only one oar – you will likely end up a great distance from your destination. A good example of not having clear distinctions is thinking we are hungry when we are, instead, emotionally upset. Eating doesn't solve the problem, and we go in reverse direction down the Path of Wellness to someplace else!

Along the Path of Wellness, somewhat near its end, is the Lake of Reflection. When you gaze into the lake you find the image of the wise Alchemist gazing back – and it is *you*. It is here, at the Lake, that you learn about the intrinsic powers you possess. First of all, you learn that an Alchemist of Experience simply takes what they learn about themselves and applies it in ways that produce pleasant experiences. It's pretty basic stuff, but most of us forget how to do it as we grow into adulthood.

At the Lake, you also learn that you will become a highly skilled Alchemist as you continue to build an ever-deepening understanding of human experience. Most importantly, the Alchemist learns that joy is always in the direction of their inspired future. Fulfillment resides only in aligned direction to your Grand Mystery; everything else turns out to be distraction!

The Path of Wellness comes to an intersection where you must choose to go either left, to The Bog of Negative Thought, or proceed right to Future's Landing. Future's Landing is a place where you might choose to contemplate your direction, reflect on your Grand Mystery, or perhaps just rest before continuing on to the Path of Inspiration. Most people, unaware of the gravity of their decision, unwittingly choose to go left toward negative thought – each for their own personal reason – but the Alchemist of Experience is buoyed by truth and curiosity.

Finding the Knapsack beside the bench at Future's Landing (with your name on it), you open it up to find each of the Alchemist's Tools especially designed for you. The Alchemist's Measure, the Language of Well-Being, and the Radar Instrument (Debris Wiper) will keep you focused on your travels. You must use these tools in the here and now to see through to today – identifying conditioned emotions and aged mythologies. You will never make it to your Grand Mystery if you continually focus on the "there and then," looking for an inspired future in the rubble of the past.

Part way down the Path of Inspiration is the oak tree at the edge of the Meadow of Wholeness. Your time in the Meadow provides an unusually vivid experience of your feeling patterns as they arise, ebb, and resolve. You are beginning to experience life from deep within your "here-and-now" consciousness. It is becoming easier to encounter life directly from native feeling, and reassuring to know that even difficult feelings will resolve to an uplifted state of mind. Isn't it good to know how well your body, mind, spirit, and environment work together, allowing your travels to broaden and your life to unfold?

Continuing on the Path of Inspiration, you come upon the Wellspring of Inspiration at the base of a steep ravine where many depleted travelers pass by you, returning from their journeys. The ravine leads to a twenty-foot-tall wall of roots and tangles that you must climb to continue your Quest. However, this is where the Golem, the evil monster of your childhood mythology, lays in hiding waiting to nip at your heels and drag you back into The Bog. Your knowledge of the mythological Golem now allows you to brush him aside with the Debris Wiper and "disappear" him as you travel forward. You know the Golem is no more real than the phantoms under your bed as a child – they simply don't exist along your journey.

The "Bench of Reflection," actually just a large horizontal tree root that looks much like a bench, overlooks a Garden where you see your yet-to-be-companion, the Dancer, engaged in the Dance of Inspiration. This is a perfect place to learn how to welcome inspiration into your consciousness and nurture it until your ideas blossom and take root. Here you learn how important the Dance of Inspiration is and how easily the Alchemists of Experience can empty their cluttered minds and imagine the lives they yearn for. With a little quiet time to empty your mind, and a comfortable space in which to think and dance, you can allow your inspiration to emerge and take root.

In the Alchemist's Garden are curious stakes with seedling packets attached to each, inviting you to plant them when you know what they are. By now you know that those seedlings are the five most important things in your life that you want to nurture and grow, that anchor you in your journey and are the beneficiaries of all that you love and all that you know. These seedlings are always a part of your journey, whether they be family, career, or forever adventures. They blossom both inside your heart and outside in the world.

The four Terraces, which begin just beyond your seedlings and reach high above the Alchemist's Garden, form four distinct levels of creative consciousness. The World of the Manifest begins at the boundary of your Garden and represents the level of awareness we are in during much of our daily activities. This level holds our day-to-day consciousness when we go to work, visit with friends and colleagues, and raise our families. Most of our days are spent in the world of "doing" in the physical world. It is also where we experience our immediate Native Feelings and Thoughts as they arise in here-and-now experience.

Directly above the World of the Manifest is the World of Mastery. This is the territory of our emotions, our drive to succeed, our depth of feeling. It is the indwelling of the heart and the fire behind our passions. In the World of Mastery, we hone our skills of relationship, learn our trades, and strive to balance our emotions and our drive. In the World of Mastery, we strive for balance and excellence and make corrections to any mythologies that may be lingering. Sometimes we find our Golem in this Terrace, and just as we believe we are about to achieve a great success (whether in a relationship or in our endeavors), the Golem will try to tug us back into the Bog of Negative Thought. The World of Mastery is a challenging and rewarding territory – and it is the place we bring our inspirations to life.

As our energies rise upward, we arrive at the World of Discernment, where we balance loving-kindness with discipline, where we weigh and measure right from wrong, good from bad, and where we develop ethical values and our sense of morality. When we are able to find balance, we also find beauty; we discover the abundance of all that is good and appreciation of the very nature of our lives.

At the top of the heights rests the World of Creative Reality. This Terrace is closest to the intersection of "all-that-is": our pinnacle of wisdom and understanding. This is an often wildly creative and vibrant state of consciousness and often offers us great calm and solace in a storm. This highly sensitive state of conscious awareness is available to us always, but to discover our inspired lives we must learn to be still and experience the quietude that launches our creativity, our deepest inspirations. From all that we have become over decades of travels, and with the wisdom we have gathered, we are able to see with ever-increasing clarity into the future that inspires us. We intuit, we know, and we move forward toward our Grand Mystery.t

The Guidebook

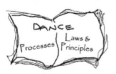

The Quagmire has its own set of physical (or mechanical) processes and laws through which it operates. To the untrained eye, life can appear all haphazard and random; but to the eyes of

the Alchemist of Experience, the orderliness of it all appears to be a great cosmic dance.

The *Process of Inspiration*, in its quiet beauty, invites us to become internally quiet, to quell our monkey minds, calm our chattering brains, and let go of our mental control. These are the steps of the Dance of Inspiration. From our internal emptiness inspiration will spontaneously arise – every time. It may be small inspiration – like go get some ice cream – or it could be the next discovery or innovation that will change the world. Inspiration comes in all sizes and they are all gems of the universe. Pick the ones that steal your heart, capture your thoughts, and beg persistent curiosity. Revel in those gems; let them grow and blossom in their detail. Nurture them, dance them about in your heart and in your mind. Plant your favorites in the Alchemist's Garden.

The second process which allows us to live into our inspired lives is the *Process of Creation*, or the Dance of Four Worlds. As Alchemists in Training we first learn the Dance of Four Worlds starting in the World of the Manifest and dance our way up through the Terraces as we gain awareness in each of four worlds until we reach the World of Creative Reality. The dance from the Manifest up to Creative reality is how we learn about ourselves and our different levels of conscious awareness. This is where we begin; by dancing from the bottom of the Terraces to the top.

However, once we become aware of our levels of consciousness, and learn how to distinguish between them, we can begin to master the Process of Creation where we actively turn our inspiration into reality. The Process of Creation begins in the World of Creative Reality where we build out our ideas from concept to formation; as we contribute them into the World of the Manifest. We live into our inspired lives by dancing from the top Terrace down into our realized dreams.

Four Worlds Choreography

Inspiration

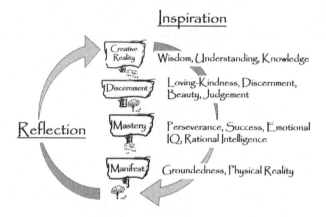

Wisdom, Understanding, Knowledge

Loving-Kindness, Discernment, Beauty, Judgement

Perseverance, Success, Emotional IQ, Rational Intelligence

Groundedness, Physical Reality

Reflection

These two concepts of learning about ourselves (*reflection* – bottom to top) and living into our inspired lives (*inspiration* – top to bottom) are critical concepts. It is important to gain proficiency in both – you will use them equally throughout your journey.

Along with Dancing in the Four Worlds are the basic physical laws and principles that accompany the dance. The laws and principles can be used as a sort of "rulebook" letting you know the depth of flexibility you have as you move about in the Four Worlds. They also let you know when you are attempting the impossible, or making significant mistakes in your choreography. How you choreograph your dance is an art. Every dance is unique; the more you practice dancing in the Four Worlds, the better you become.

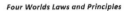

Four Worlds Laws and Principles

Law #1 – *Each World has a unique Purpose - The Principle of Consciousness asserts that our states of consciousness shift to achieve the purpose of each world.*

Law #2 – *Creation is iterative. The Principle of Movement asserts that we are free to move within a single world's energies, or between the Four Worlds in any order we choose.*

Law #3 – *All questions have an answer. The Principle of Dual Nature asserts that our observer and the selves we observe work together without error.*

Law #4 – *Each World as its Boundaries – The Principle of Permeability asserts that boundaries between worlds must be permeable to achieve wellbeing.*

Law #5 – *Progress is constant. The Principle of Evidence of Success asserts that progress is always present in the direction you have chosen.*

Law #6 – *Communities are a shared Creation – The Principle of Community asserts that communities create themselves through the consciousness of its individual participants.*

Frontier Adventure

We each have our own "Grand Mystery" to explore during our lifetime – and perhaps into the next. Our Grand Mystery shows itself through those things we yearn to know about and that we would love to dedicate much of our time to in exploration. What has undauntingly tickled your imagination throughout your life? What calls you to action, to explore and expand?

Some experts urge us to find a purpose, set a goal, and get going. But life doesn't really work so neatly. As we look across our decades, we find we have many open questions about life, about how the universe works and how we work. Some of our questions are persistent, and there is usually one "whopper," one Grand Mystery, that we set out explore during our lifetime.

By nature, we are curious human beings, we love challenge, and better yet we love a good mystery. We want to know what eludes us, we search for answers, we follow our hearts, and – knowingly or not – live into our desires. There is nothing better than living on the cutting edge of what excites, and nothing more fulfilling than discovering answers and sharing them with others.

We also love to contribute, to be a source of knowledge, love, and inspiration for others, to have participated in something of importance in the world, and to allow our contributions to take root.

We seek to explore our Grand Mystery and live our lives with a sense of adventure and achievement. We create our lives in order that we may thrive and provide the treasures of our exploration to others.

Seek – Create – Give
A radical new paradigm for living a meaningful life.

Can we really devote a lifetime to seeking our Grand Mystery? Has anyone ever succeeded? Do we have role models?

✦ Albert Einstein wanted to solve the mysteries of the universe and share them with the world; and he did.

✦ Indira Gandhi, India's first female Prime Minister, wanted to invigorate and strengthen India; and she did.

✦ Elon Musk wants to change the world and humanity; and he is.

✦ My son's fourth-grade teacher wanted to explore the world of mathematics and share her joy of learning with her students; and she did.

✦ My mother wanted to explore the depths of independence and share the treasure of inspired living; and she did.

So many people live their lives out of a sense of obligation rather than *living into what inspires.* What would change if you could follow your dreams, seek out the mysteries of your life, and share your treasures with those you love? That is ultimately the pot of gold at the end of rainbow that will fulfill us and give our lives depth of meaning.

There is much to learn about being *you.* Discover and embrace your own Grand Mysteries, ask the Big Questions, truly grasp what it is that you yearn for. Graciously allow the way of your inspiration to propel you forward and witness the "enfold-ment" of what will emerge next. All questions will be answered simply because they have been asked; relentlessly live into the power of your inspiration and give *Your Book of Life Past* a twist that will be forever remembered.

Your Alchemist's Knapsack is now freshly packed with everything you need to get started on your travels. Here is a blessing from me to you:

For all the wisdom and understanding
you hold in your heart;
Live always with compassion and discernment
knowing that you matter;
Acknowledging all that you have lived
through in your life and all that you have
brought forth into today;
And for all that you will bring forward into all
of your tomorrows –
I wish you grace in the journey ahead.

~

Quietly, you nestle into a quiet spot in your Alchemist's Garden alongside a shallow pond. The air is warm and pungent with the sweet smell of fresh grasses and wild jasmine. Life is teeming all about you and your seedlings look strong and well nourished. You pleasure at watching them grow, and you reflect back on all that you've learned since embarking on this Frontier Adventure.

"Let's go," whispers the dancer into your ear. By now you are familiar with your dancing sojourner!

Hoping to capture a memorable reflection of the two of you – like staring at a best-of-times family photo – you gaze into the pond and see only yourself.

"Inspiration calls," urges the Dancer of Four Worlds

Suddenly you understand: The Dancer is you, and your Grand Mystery awaits.

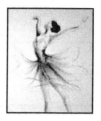

Alchemist's Practice

You have before you a Grand Mystery and all the knowledge and tools to get you started on your **Frontier Adventure**. You are becoming a capable **Alchemist** – you now understand that Alchemy is taking what you learn about yourself and applying it in a way that causes you pleasure as you **choose** to journey in the *right direction* toward your **Grand Mystery** and its **Treasure**.

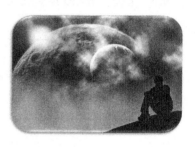

There are two skills the Alchemist of Experience uses that most people don't exercise:

1. they build an ever-deepening understanding of human experience and...

2. they make clear adjustments in themselves that are in *alignment* with the *futures* that inspire them.

Before continuing on your journey, reflect on some of key ideas you have discovered that will help keep you on track.

~

1. What is your Grand Mystery? What Big Questions are you
   currently exploring?

   Grand Mystery   Big Questions

   _____   _____

   _____   _____

   _____   _____

   _____   _____

2. What is your Treasure you will bring into the world?

   _____

   _____

   _____

   _____

3. What "seedlings" have you planted in your Alchemist's Garden?
   "What's Next" for each?

   "Seedlings"   "What's Next?"

   _____   _____

   _____   _____

   _____   _____

   _____   _____

4. Have you met your Golem? What was the experience?

_____

_____

_____

_____

5. What are the greatest challenges that you have today standing between you and your Grand Mystery? What skills do you need to practice to keep you going in the *right direction*?

_____

_____

_____

_____

> And in the end, the treasures you take are equal to the choices you make.
>
> JKS Zetlan

About the Author

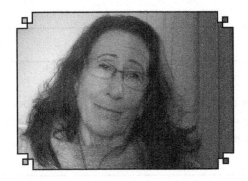

Jenifer K. S. Zetlan is a master alchemist, author, poet, and lecturer whose Treasure is helping people live inspired lives. With degrees in psychology and behavioral sciences from UCLA, she has led numerous seminars and classes in psychology, leadership, and organization in University settings and throughout many Fortune 500 companies. She has also enjoyed successful careers in psychology, aerospace, and heath care.

Jenifer has been reading, studying, and speaking in the areas of psychology, philosophy, and religion for over thirty years. She is an ardent yoga practitioner and instructor in the Bay Area.

She and her husband Andy are living into inspiration in the Bay Area.

CPSIA information can be obtained
at www.ICGtesting.com
Printed in the USA
BVOW08s1933061017
496835BV00003B/3/P